SELF-TALK
FOR
WEIGHT
LOSS

Other books by Shad Helmstetter:

WHAT TO SAY WHEN YOU TALK TO YOUR SELF
THE SELF-TALK SOLUTION
PREDICTIVE PARENTING—WHAT TO SAY WHEN YOU TALK
TO YOUR KIDS
CHOICES
FINDING THE FOUNTAIN OF YOUTH INSIDE YOURSELF
YOU CAN EXCEL IN TIME OF CHANGE

Other books by Bob Schwartz:

DIETS DON'T WORK
DIETS STILL DON'T WORK

Shad Helmstetter, Ph.D.

SELF-TALK
FOR
WEIGHT
LOSS

LOSE WEIGHT,
KEEP IT OFF, AND
NEVER DIET AGAIN

With Bob Schwartz, Ph.D.

St. Martin's Paperbacks

Published by arrangement with River Productions, Inc.

SELF-TALK FOR WEIGHT LOSS

ISBN: 0-312-95909-5

Printed in the United States of America

Breakthru Publishing hardcover edition published in 1994
St. Martin's Paperbacks edition/May 1996

10 9 8 7 6 5 4 3 2 1

This book is lovingly dedicated to Bonnie Elise Helmstetter.
—S.H.

To the love of my life, Leah.
—R.M.S.

Contents

Introduction
To The Most Important Person In The World
By Dr. Bob Schwartz

Part I
How Self-Talk Works. 1

Chapter One
Making It Simple, Keeping It Clear. 2

Chapter Two
The Truth Is, Diets *Don't* Work!. 5

Chapter Three
The Computer That Controls Your Weight. 13

Chapter Four
What If You're Not The Problem?. 20

Chapter Five
The Strongest Program Always Wins. 28

Chapter Six
Programs About Dieting, Exercise, And Eating 34

Chapter Seven
Seven Programs That Control Your Weight. 41

Chapter Eight
Who's Voting On Your Weight? 53

Chapter Nine
Changing Your Programs—
Changing Your Weight. 63

Chapter Ten
The Most "Natural" Solution We've Found. 70

Part II
Self-Talk Techniques For
Natural Weight Control 82

Chapter Eleven
How To Practice Self-Talk For Weight-Loss 83

Chapter Twelve
Self-Talk Technique #1
Monitoring Your Own Self-Talk 94

Chapter Thirteen
Self-Talk Technique #2
Turning Your Self-Talk Around 102

Chapter Fourteen
Self-Talk Technique #3
The Self-Talk "Workout". 112

Chapter Fifteen
Self-Talk Technique #4
Practicing Situational Self-Talk. 124

Chapter Sixteen
Self-Talk Technique #5
Listening To Self-Talk 131

Chapter Seventeen
Winning The Seven Greatest Battles
Of Weight-Loss. 145

Chapter Eighteen
Getting Your Self-Talk Right 162

Part III
"Naturally Thin" Techniques
To Use With Your Self-Talk 177

Chapter Nineteen
Beginning To Act Like A "Naturally Thin" Person. . 178

Chapter Twenty
Listening To Your Emotions 190

Chapter Twenty-One
A Taste Of The Thin Life 195

Part IV
Putting It All Together 205

Chapter Twenty-Two
20 Key Questions About
Self-Talk For Weight-Loss 206

Chapter Twenty-Three
Self-Talk And Setting Goals 222

Chapter Twenty-Four
The Three Stages Of Self-Talk—
You've Got A Lot To Look Forward To 240

Chapter Twenty-Five
The Second Stage Of Self-Talk:
Watching It Work 254

Chapter Twenty-Six
The Final Stage Of Self-Talk:
The Change 259

SELF-TALK
FOR
WEIGHT
LOSS

Introduction
To The Most Important Person In The World

By Bob Schwartz, Ph.D.

A number of years ago, after I had written *Diets Don't Work*, and *Diets Still Don't Work*, I began hearing about the exciting new work that was being done in the field called "Self-Talk." After writing my first books and appearing on hundreds of talk shows and television programs, I was conducting special training classes around the United States for people who wanted help controlling their weight, and I knew I had found most of the answers to the problem.

Dr. Shad Helmstetter, a Ph.D. in motivational psychology who pioneered the field of Self-Talk, had written several best-selling books on the subject, including *What To Say When You Talk To Your Self*, and *The Self-Talk Solution*.

Finally, I had the opportunity to hear Dr. Helmstetter speak in person at a seminar program he was conducting on the subject of Self-Talk for weight-loss. I was fascinated with the whole idea of using Self-Talk with my clients, workshop attendees, and my book readers, and I knew Dr. Helmstetter's work could help those who were interested in permanent weight control. As it turned out, Dr. Helmstetter had found and perfected the missing piece to the puzzle.

For over fifteen years, Dr. Helmstetter had been researching and developing the concept of changing mental programs to create long-term changes in habits and behavior. With Self-Talk, Dr. Helmstetter had discovered a major breakthrough in how programming works, but he also had another winning attribute—Dr. Helmstetter was able to make the concept of Self-Talk come *alive*; he made it so simple that anyone could do it. As you will find in the pages that follow, he knows how to talk in a language that everyone can understand.

This book brings together, for the first time ever, some of the best proven concepts and ideas that I have used and taught for more than a decade, with what I believe to be the most important *final* step in permanent weight control we have ever found—*Self-Talk*—the final piece of the puzzle.

In the following pages, Dr. Helmstetter shows you how Self-Talk works, and what *really* causes the weight problems in the first place. Then, in the "how-to" section, we'll give you specific techniques that you can put into practice starting immediately.

If you are one of the many thousands of people Dr. Helmstetter or I have instructed in one of our seminar programs, who have asked us to put the very best Self-Talk and *"naturally thin"* techniques together in one easy-to-follow guide—here it is.

This book is also written for the millions of individuals who would like to look better, feel better, and get in control of their weight—and their lives—*permanently*. We believe that you are the most important person in the world.

This book is for you.

Bob Schwartz, Ph.D.
Houston, Texas

Part I
How Self-Talk Works

Chapter One
Making It Simple, Keeping It Clear

After losing my fight against weight for many years, I made the decision to try something called "Self-Talk." By using Self-Talk techniques and changing the old mental "programs" that had caused the weight in the first place, I lost fifty-eight pounds—and kept it off. It was clear that the techniques of Self-Talk worked. I weigh less now than I did then. And I have never been on a "diet" since.

When I first began doing my early pioneering work in Self-Talk, long before I wrote my first of six books on the subject (and long before I lost the weight), I don't think I ever considered that this new concept would end up changing my own life. I was researching the field of motivational psychology, and I was interested only in what makes us do what we do, and what *stops* us from doing what is best for us. It was during that research that I discovered what we now call Self-Talk.

For over fifteen years now, I have continued to study this amazing concept of human behavior. During that time, we've learned a lot about Self-Talk and how it works.

Through medical research, we have learned that the human brain operates like a powerful, personal computer—and like that computer, you and I receive programs that become permanent "pathways" in our brains. And as we now know, those are the programs we end up living out.

Your self-esteem, your attitudes, your beliefs about anything, your motivation, and even your weight, end up being determined by the programs you carry around with you.

If you are like most of us, what you weigh right now is based almost entirely on the programs you already have. And until recently, we understood almost nothing about programs, or what to do about them. We thought, *"That's just the way I am. I was born that way, and that's the way I was destined to be."*

It's time to set the record straight. Medical, neurological, and behavioral research has shown that not only can we learn how to erase or replace the programs we got, but we can literally change our *lives* when we change the program paths in our brains.

You will find that learning and using the Self-Talk techniques isn't complicated, and it isn't difficult to do. Anyone can do it, and most of the techniques don't take any extra time.

Yet these techniques are among the strongest and most effective we have ever found to help people change their weight naturally and permanently. If you have a problem with weight, of any kind, what you learn in this book will help.

COMBINING THE TECHNIQUES OF "SELF-TALK" AND BEING "NATURALLY THIN"

As Dr. Bob Schwartz pointed out in the introduction, this book gives you a combination of techniques to follow. Dr. Schwartz' work has helped literally thousands of people with weight problems. By themselves, his techniques for helping people become "naturally thin" have made a profound difference in people's lives. Combined with Self-Talk, those techniques now offer you a lifetime of success and satisfaction, instead of years of fighting food and gaining weight.

As you will discover, being naturally thin is not only possible, but you have a *very* good chance of reaching that goal yourself. With the right Self-Talk to help you *change* the programs that caused the weight problem in the *first* place, that's a goal you could keep for the rest of your life.

Chapter Two
The Truth Is, Diets *Don't* Work!

Why can't we find a diet that works? What goes wrong? What stops it from working?

For years I watched too many good people get started at reaching a goal—and then stop, put it off, or fail. It wasn't that they didn't *want* to reach the goal; it was more like something else kept getting in the way.

I watched my struggles with my own waistline as I inched upward from size 32 to beyond size 40. For me, that represented an increase of over 50 pounds—and even more deplorable, a *downward* spiral of my self-esteem. And it seemed the more I tried to *do* about it, the more diets I tried, the less successful I was. "Something *else*" was stopping me.

WE KNOW IT'S TRUE: *DIETS DON'T WORK!*

And it wasn't just stopping *me*. The more I studied, the more I saw the exact same failure mechanism at work in lives all around me. Most people (about 97%) spend more time fighting failure than they spend enjoying success.

In his bestselling book *Diets Still Don't Work*, and in

his public seminars, Dr. Bob Schwartz shares the story of how he proved conclusively that diets don't work, when he helped people in his health clubs safely *gain* weight by repeatedly starting and stopping a standard *"reducing"* diet until they had gained all the weight they wanted. He proved that diets work in a way, though—they work in *reverse*, because of the cycle of lowering metabolism they can create in the body.

Dr. Schwartz also tells about his own struggles with weight. Here is his story in his own words:

"Between the ages of thirty and forty, I had lost over 2,000 pounds from dieting—not all at once, of course, but on successive diets. During this period I owned twenty-six health clubs in the west and southwest. I had been on a hundred different diets during that ten-year period, and was successful every time at reaching my weight-loss goal. But my weight always returned once I stopped dieting.

"The problem was that every time I lost my extra 20 to 40 pounds, it was taking longer and longer to get the weight off. And, every time I gained my weight back, it came back faster and faster.

"I reached the end of my rope one Monday morning when I got up and started to go to work. I had been on a weekend-long, out-of-control, non-stop eating binge, and I found that I could not button even my largest size pants.

"I was terrified. Who wouldn't be? I owned a chain of health clubs, and chubby weight-loss experts are not very popular. What was even worse was that I had to call in and say that I wasn't coming to work. Have you ever had to call in 'fat?'

"I was stumped. I knew everything about exercise, diet, and nutrition, and yet I could no longer lose weight and keep it off. I had become more and more obsessive

6

about eating instead of less and less. I was a success in every area of my life except weight control. My overeating and extra weight seemed to invalidate everything else I had accomplished.

"How could someone who had the willpower to figure out every other problem that life had thrown at him not be able to control his weight and eating? What was I doing wrong?"

THE DIFFERENCE BETWEEN "*NATURALLY* THIN" AND "*ARTIFICIALLY* THIN"

Dr. Schwartz and I were approaching the same dilemma from slightly different points of view: he, from the standpoint of a diet and exercise expert, and I, from the area of motivational psychology. And we both came up with the same conclusion, independently: some people can lose weight and keep it off—or never seem to have a problem with it in the first place—and for others, it is a never-ending battle.

Each of us, in our own research, then decided on the same next step: to take a look at the differences between those two groups of people.

Here is what Dr. Schwartz discovered:

"For twenty years I had been learning everything that *overweight* people knew about losing weight. I had been studying the wrong people. It was as if I had been studying how poor people try to get rich. If you want to get rich and stay rich, you don't study poor people. Even if you were only a little bit smart, you would study rich people who had become rich and stayed rich.

"At first I talked to the thin people who had at one time

been overweight. I limited this group to those who had kept their weight off for at least five years. But studying people who lost their weight and kept it off by dieting— that 1/2 of 1 percent of dieters—proved to be a dead end.

"These *'artificially thin people,'* as I began to call them, seemed to have compulsive personalities. They used to overeat compulsively—now they dieted, counted calories, worried about gaining their weight back, and underate compulsively. They spent all of their energy, time, and attention on what they ate or what they didn't eat . . . on how much they gained or how much they lost . . . on how much they had exercised or in worrying that they hadn't done enough. Their compulsive behavior drove people around them crazy, and was not the way I wanted to live the rest of my life.

"Then I decided that I would begin to study *naturally thin* people. This idea had not occurred to me before, because I had thought that all naturally thin people stayed thin because their bodies burned food faster than other people's bodies. I was convinced that it was their high metabolism rate which should be given credit. But what if the answer was something else? What if they knew something that I did not know—something that I might have forgotten? After all, I too had been a naturally thin person until age thirty.

"In studying naturally thin people, I learned that they do four fundamental things when they eat that overweight people don't.

1. They don't eat unless their body is *hungry*.

2. They eat *exactly* what they want—*exactly* what will satisfy them.

3. They don't eat unconsciously; they *enjoy* every bite of what they are eating, and they are aware of the effect the food is having on their bodies.

4. They stop eating when their bodies are no longer

hungry.

"I knew that if I could just figure out _how_ the naturally thin people avoided overeating without dieting or depriving themselves of whatever they wanted, I would have the secret to losing weight and keeping it off."

Dr. Schwartz brings up a vital point: that in order to win the weight-loss battle, we have to understand why some people overeat—and some people don't.

WHY PEOPLE EAT—
AND WHAT MAKES THEM _OVEREAT_

Take a moment and look through the following list of the most common reasons people give for why they eat.

As you read through the list, see if you can tell what all of these reasons have in common:

21 REASONS PEOPLE SAY THEY EAT:

1. _"I eat when I'm bored."_
2. _"I eat when I'm hungry. . .and I'm always hungry."_
3. _"I eat when I've had a bad day."_
4. _"I eat because I have a craving for chocolate."_
5. _"I eat when I worry."_
6. _"I eat when I'm watching TV."_
7. _"I have to keep putting something in my mouth."_
8. _"I eat more every time I plan to go on a diet."_
9. _"I eat when I'm frustrated."_
10. _"I eat to make the cook happy."_
11. _"I eat to reward myself."_
12. _"I eat when I'm unhappy."_

13. *"I eat to make myself feel better."*
14. *"I eat because I just like to eat."*
15. *"I eat because I can't lose weight anyway."*
16. *"I eat because it's the only pleasure I have."*
17. *"I eat because I don't have the will power not to."*
18. *"I eat because I'm lonely."*
19. *"I eat to feel secure."*
20. *"If I don't eat it, it will just go to waste."*
21. *"I eat it because it's there."*

Perhaps you can add a few reasons of your own, or reasons you've heard others give for wanting to eat.

Did you notice what all of the reasons on that list have in common? Not *one* of the reasons given for eating mentioned *nutrition*.

Outside of the human species, all animals in their natural state eat *only* for the purpose of *maintaining health and nutrition*. And that is the way *naturally thin* people eat—but not the way overweight or "artificially thin" people eat.

We can take that rule one step further: The reason people eat is for nutrition. The reason they *overeat* (which includes eating the wrong food) has little or nothing to do with nutrition—or with food—at all. We *eat* to fulfill the needs of the body. We *overeat* to fulfill the needs of the *mind*.

WHERE IT ALL BEGINS

To find out where the problem starts, I decided to begin by taking a look into that amazing place where we live our entire lives; the place where our personality resides, where our attitudes take root, our choices dwell, and every step we take is formed: the human brain.

In studying all kinds of people, I, too, noticed some distinct differences between overweight people, "artificially thin" people, and "naturally thin" people. Among the many conclusions I came to was that the primary difference between them was not in *"what"* they were eating (or curiously, even how much they ate). It was in what was going on in their *minds* at the precise moment they took each bite of food.

Each of the individuals who was *consciously* aware of trying to keep weight off was, moment by moment, getting either a "yes" vote or a "no" vote on each bite he or she was taking. It was as if a silent supervisor, like a movie director sitting in their internal control center somewhere "upstairs," was monitoring each bite and saying, *"Oh, go ahead, take the bite, it won't hurt you,"* or *"You really shouldn't have any more,"* or *"Well, okay, you've been pretty good today, have one more piece of cake,"* or *"Absolutely not!"* or *"Go ahead, eat it—it will make you feel better."*

And it became clear that the directions those people were getting from somewhere in their own minds were as real as if someone was actually sitting right there with them, telling them what to do, sometimes scolding, sometimes praising, but *always* directing the show.

I also observed that the people who were *not* troubled by weight problems—the *"naturally thin"* people— seemed to have almost *no* silent directions about food, coming from and going to their control centers.

Never once did I see someone come up to the table and physically force someone else to take a bite. The struggles I observed were never *external*; they were always fought *within*—and very quickly. Instant, ten-second "wars of will" were fought—and won or lost—dozens of

11

times at a single meal. Most of the individuals were not even aware the battles were being fought. And all those little wars were fought in the individual's own *brain*.

It would be there, somewhere inside that brain, that I knew I would find the answer I was looking for.

Chapter Three
The Computer That Controls Your Weight

Recently, the people whose job it is to study the human brain have learned more about *why* we do what we do, than was known throughout all of history prior to that time.

What they have learned has unlocked some very important secrets that have to do with our weight. Because it will help you to understand what they have learned, I will give you a brief overview of the discoveries they've made.

YOUR BRAIN IS A POWERFUL COMPUTER—AND YOUR "COMPUTER" CONTROLS YOUR WEIGHT

Remember that the neuroscientists who are making these discoveries are not people who are trying to find the answers to weight-loss or self-motivation. What they *are* interested in is how the brain actually works.

Most of the recent breakthroughs in mind/brain research have been made possible by new computer technology. The new "medical imaging technology" allows researchers, for the first time, to look into the human brain *while it is operating*. Now they can watch us think, *while we're thinking*—and a whole lot more.

The researchers discovered that in many ways, your brain operates much like a powerful, personal computer. There are differences, of course, but in many respects, even the most powerful computers we have today are patterned after the *human* computers that created them.

Many of the functions of the brain can be compared to specific parts and functions of a computer. Most computers have keyboards, video screens, and floppy disks. We have learned that you and I have similar parts. Here are a few of the computer-like parts that *you* have that help you get through each day:

YOUR COMPUTER "KEYBOARD"—
YOUR FIVE SENSES

You were born with your own personal computer keyboard. On a computer, the keyboard is what we use to type in new messages or commands—or anything we want to "program" into the computer. In us, the computer keyboard is our five senses. It is through our five senses that we get all of the messages that are programmed into us.

Imagine that you were born holding your keyboard out to the world in front of you. If you could have talked at the time, you might have said something like:

"Here, Mom; here, Dad; here, world—I don't know how to do this yet, so I need some help typing in my programs. First I need you to type in who I am, and what direction I should go. That's the direction I will follow. Along the way, I need you to type in some values, and some strength, and some courage and some integrity, so I'll be able to follow the path you set for me. But most of all, along with the life you have given me and the love you will share with me along the way . . . I need you to tell me how far I will go . . . and that is exactly how far I will go, and what I will do, with this life that is in front of me. *Would you please program me so that I can live up to my full potential . . .* would you show me who I *can* become?"

And our parents, and our teachers, and our brothers and sisters, and all the other people around us did not know that on top of our keyboard was a bright yellow diamond-shaped sign that said, *"Warning! Anything you type into this child's computer keyboard will be stored for life—and acted on as though it is true."* They didn't know; and had they known, they would never have given us most of the programs we got.

Look at what we've discovered about our own "mental computers" and the programs *you* have been receiving:

Since the moment you were born, every message you have ever received has been programmed into your personal computer—and stored permanently in your brain.

That means that *every* message you have ever received—everything that has ever been said to you, everything you have ever seen or experienced, everything you have ever done, everything you have ever said, everything you have thought consciously, and even those thoughts you didn't know you were thinking—*every single message you have ever gotten, from any source, has been programmed into your brain, and stored there permanently.*

YOUR "FLOPPY DISK"—
YOUR SUBCONSCIOUS MIND

The researchers have also learned that when you were born you received a "floppy disk," like the magnetic disk used to record new programs or information in computers. In your computer brain, however, that storage disk is called your "subconscious mind."

What we call the subconscious mind is not a specific place in the brain. It is a facility that works throughout many areas of the brain. We have also learned that the subconscious mind follows specific *rules*—and these rules are important to the programs that affect your success in dealing with weight, right now:

Rule 1. Every program you have ever received—from any source—has been stored permanently in your subconscious mind.

Rule 2. The subconscious mind—that part of the brain that stores the programs—does not know the difference between something that is TRUE and something that is FALSE.

The subconscious mind is not the same part of the brain that you are reading with and thinking with right now. We're talking here about the part of your brain that stores all of the programs you receive. Just like the floppy disk in your computer at home or at the office, the subconscious mind does not know the difference between something that is right or wrong, bad or good, positive or negative, harmful or helpful. It just stores the information, and acts on the programs it receives.

Could you walk up to your computer keyboard at home

16

or at the office and type something into it that is not *true*? Of course you could. Would your computer care? No, it wouldn't. In most computers it wouldn't make any difference at all. (Otherwise we couldn't write novels.)

Your computer simply accepts and stores anything you program into it. In the same way, so does your subconscious mind. That's what it was designed to do.

YOUR PROGRAMS DETERMINE YOUR WEIGHT

Imagine that the subconscious mind (in everyone) is, at all times, busily storing—*permanently*—*all* of the programs it is receiving. Then imagine hearing some parent say, *"Susie, you're going to grow up to be chubby, just like your Aunt Harriet!"* Or how about the little boy being told, *"Timmy, you'd lose your head if wasn't screwed on."* Or the hopeful young girl who is told, *"Jennifer, I wouldn't try out for cheerleading if I were you, sweetheart . . . you're not really cut out for that."*

We can only imagine that somewhere deep down inside is a child's dream that would like to shout, *"I won't have a chance at being healthy if you program me that way,"* or *"Thanks, Dad— now I know I won't be organized,"* or *"I know I won't be good at cheerleading— you've told me that before!"*

The programs we receive, good or bad, turn out to be a lot more important than we might have thought. The reason they are so important is because of the next rule we learned about the subconscious mind:

Rule 3. The subconscious mind is designed to always act on the strongest programs it has.

The programs *you* have right now that are the strongest are the programs that are actually in control. You don't even have to know what programs they are, or where they came from.

Rule 4. The subconscious mind is designed to get more of (or duplicate) the programs it already has that are the strongest.

The saying, "like attracts like" is true of our programming. Whatever programs we already have, we consciously and *unconsciously* seek out or attract more programs just like them. Instead of constantly getting rid of programs that might work against us, we *duplicate* them.

FOLLOWING THE RULES

When it comes to the human brain—and what we call the *"mind"*—some would have us believe we're dealing with some kind of mystical, other-worldly magic. We're not. We are dealing with a biological organ, one that we are beginning to learn a great deal about.

A number of years ago we didn't know much about the human heart, so medical researchers studied it. They recognized that the human heart is a biological organ, and as such, it has some very specific physical rules to follow. Your heart, and mine, will follow those rules from its first beat to its last.

Because we studied the heart, we now know a lot more about it. We know how to feed the heart differently than we used to. We know more about how to exercise it properly. We can even fix it now when something goes wrong, and sometimes we can even replace it when it breaks. It doesn't make any difference to my heart itself if I don't understand that, or if I don't believe what the doctors have learned about how it works. My heart will just continue to follow its rules, from its first beat to its last.

In the same way, medical researchers studied the human brain. They recognized that it, too, is an organ—and it, too, has certain specific rules it was designed to follow. Like the heart, the brain does not care if we understand its rules or even believe in them. It will simply go on following those unbreakable rules *exactly as it was designed to*—from our first moment of life until our last.

Your own brain, *right now*, is doing exactly what it was designed to do. It is following its rules. It is storing programs—about you—and acting them out, whether those programs are "true"—or not.

Chapter Four

What If You're Not The Problem?

In my first book on the subject of Self-Talk, I included the estimate that during the first eighteen years of life, the average individual is told *"no,"* or what he or she *cannot* do, more than *148,000* times.

I now believe that is a *low* estimate. In fact, isn't it true that a lot of the messages we got while we were growing up were messages that were never said to us out loud? What about "that look" we got at the dinner table? Or how about the test papers that came back from the teacher with the number *wrong* at the top instead of the number *right*? Or the parent who didn't show up for some event that perhaps he or she should have attended? We received hundreds of thousands of messages, both spoken and unspoken. However many programs we received, it doesn't take too close a look to know many of those programs were the wrong kind.

The question here is not whether you or I received a hundred thousand programs like those, or a half a million. The truth is that *all* of the programs you received, regardless what they were, are still with you today—and those programs that are the strongest are the programs that are in control—right now.

77% OF ALL OUR PROGRAMS MAY BE FALSE

Behavioral researchers have estimated that in the average individual, *as much as 77% of all our programs are false.* That means that as much as *three-fourths* of all of our programs may be *wrong,* counter-productive, or work against us. And that's if we grew up with a reasonably positive home life! What if that estimate is correct?

I have met people who I believe may have as much as ninety or ninety-five percent of their programs working against them. All you have to do is look at them in their endless struggles: fighting their way through a life fraught only with problems and self-created misadventure, following a path that is so poorly laid that they literally have no idea where they're headed. That is a life that is not working. That is an individual whose programs have failed.

Fortunately, most of us have been blessed with some programs that are better than that. But what about the programs we have that *are* the wrong kind? We now know that we don't even have to know *what* our programs are or *where* we got them. Our computer doesn't care. We just follow the programs we have that are the strongest—even if we don't know they exist.

A LOOK AT WHAT ONE PROGRAM CAN DO

I was on a radio talk show in Chicago when a man named Jim called in to the show. Jim told me, "Dr. Helmstetter, during the last fifteen minutes while you were talking about how the brain gets programmed, and

21

those programs are permanent and determine everything about us—while you were explaining that, I discovered the reason for a problem that has been destroying my life for the past thirty-six years."

"What was that?" I asked, very interested in what Jim would say next.

"While I was listening to you," Jim said, "I remembered an incident that happened to me when I was six years old . . . and it changed my life."

I asked Jim if the incident was something he could talk about on the air. He said it was—and then he told me, and the listening audience, what had happened.

"I remembered, just now, for the first time ever," Jim said, "sitting in my desk one day when I was in first grade. It was parents' visiting day at my school. And I remember sitting in my desk in my classroom, and my teacher was standing right in front of my desk. She was tall, so she was standing way above me. And right behind me, behind my right shoulder, stood my mother, and she was also very tall above me. I heard my teacher talking to my mother about me. I heard my teacher say to my mother, *'Jimmy is a slow learner; I don't think he'll ever do well in school, and I don't think he will ever go to college!'*"

Can you imagine the strength of that program? Do you suppose little Jimmy ever had to be told that same program again by that same teacher for the program to stick?

No, programs like that take off with a life of their own. Every time Jimmy went up to the blackboard to write something in front of the class—and his little classmates called him "dummy," or "stupid," or the things kids call each other—*it was the same program again.*

Or how about when Jimmy got his test papers handed back to him? Do you suppose Jimmy looked for a gold star at the top of *his* papers? Never! Not Jimmy. He wasn't cut out for that. *Again and again the program was repeated.* Day by day it got stronger and stronger.

Or how about the day when Jim was a junior in high school and over the public address system came the announcement, *"Attention, students! Tomorrow morning at ten o'clock in the gymnasium, there will be representatives from colleges and universities. All students planning on going on to college after high school be in the gymnasium at 10 o'clock sharp tomorrow morning."* Do you suppose young Jim was first in line that next morning to get down to the gymnasium to talk to someone about his future in college? I wouldn't be surprised if Jim stayed home from school that day.

I talked to Jim, now thirty-six years later, on the radio long enough to know this: He told me he has spent thirty-six years trying to graduate from *anything*! He told me that early incident had gone on to affect everything else about him. He said it had clearly determined his career path (he didn't call it a "career path"; he called it "a series of endless jobs"). He said that program definitely determined how much money he made. And he said without any doubt, that incident had started *other* programs that in time completely eroded his self-esteem. But most of all, Jim said, he recognized now that the programs that incident created had even helped determine who he chose to be his *wife*—to spend his *life* with!

And I talked to Jim long enough to know this, too: Do you think what happened to Jim's life had anything to do with his *intelligence*? It had *nothing* to do with his intelligence whatsoever! It had to do with a "gift" that he received from someone else—from a teacher in school who would never have given him that gift in the first place if she had had any *idea* of what she was *taking* from his life.

23

You may not have programs that are that disastrous, but the point is that Jim did not have to know where the programs had come from—*or that the programs were even there in the first place*. They did their job just the same.

Our programs may not be that bad, but what if 77% of our own programs are the *wrong* kind of programs?

THE PROGRAMS THAT ARE SETTING YOUR COURSE AND DIRECTION RIGHT NOW

I once suggested to my readers that they look at those programs in the same way we might look at the programs that are typed into the on-board computer on an airplane.

Let us say I invited you on an all-expenses-paid vacation for two glorious weeks in the Caribbean. It is the day of our departure, and we are at the airport, excited about our trip. Finally, they call our flight, and we gather our bags with our suntan lotion and swim fins and books to read, and begin to board the plane. Then, as we are getting on the plane, we happen to overhear the navigator whispering to the captain—and we hear him say, "Captain, we have a *problem!*"

The captain says, "What is it?" and the navigator responds, "Captain, we've just discovered that 77% of the airplane's on-board computer programs—*the programs that fly the plane*—are the *wrong* programs!"

If we heard that astonishing news, what would we do next?

We would get off the plane! If 77% of that airplane's on-board computer programs are the wrong programs, that plane is going to *crash*—or at *best* it is going to land in the wrong place. Those are the computer programs that will determine that airplane's *course, altitude, speed*, and final *destination—everything* about the journey we are about to take.

But you might say, "My programs are better than that. I don't have 77% of my life's programs that are the wrong kind." I hope that is true. But would we get on that airplane if we heard that only *50%* of its programs were the wrong programs? No, we wouldn't. What about *25%*? I would not get on that airplane, nor do I suspect would you get on that plane with me if we heard that *any* of its programs were the wrong programs.

And yet we do it every day! We get up in the morning, put our computer disk in, and leap headlong into our day. Imagine being able to hold in your hand a floppy disk that contained every single program you have right now. Now imagine tucking that disk under your arm each morning and have it immediately begin *programming* and setting up your day for you.

Instantly, the programs start to play . . . *Should I really watch my diet today? . . . No, I'll put that off until next week . . . Get organized? . . . A little later, maybe . . . Fit into just the right dress for work? . . . No, this'll have to do . . . Have a great day? . . . No, it's another blue Monday . . . Get things done today? Get on top and in control? . . . I'm not in the mood . . . !*

I'm not implying that your programs are anything like those. Your day may always get off on the right foot and stay that way. But however it goes, whatever you do— today and *every* day—you can be sure the programs you carry with you determine *your* course, your altitude, your speed, and your destination.

Your programs are designed to determine what you think and do about anything and everything, every moment. Just like with the airplane, your programs make the difference between a life that's not working quite right, and one that could be working a whole lot better—in weight and in every other area.

EVERY PROGRAM YOU HAVE EVER RECEIVED IS STILL WITH YOU

A team of medical researchers, could, right now, place you under an anesthetic, and by administering a minor electrical current to a small cluster of neurons at a precise point in your brain—you would, in that moment, *completely* recall and *relive* an experience from when you were, say, three years old at your three-year-old birthday party.

But you wouldn't just remember the experience; you would literally *be back there, then.* You would, in that instant, *completely* relive the experience. You would taste the tastes that you tasted then; you would smell the smells that were there then.

You would even be able to hear things that were said to you then that you didn't even understand at the time because you were only three years old. But you would understand them now because you would be an adult, *back* in the mind and the body of you as a three-year-old child. You would even feel the touch of the clothes that you were wearing then. You would even be able to feel the emotions that you felt on that day!

There is only *one* way those neuroscientists could bring all of that back: that is if it is *all still there.* And it *is* all still there—along with *every other* program you have ever received and carry with you today.

IT ISN'T *YOU*—IT'S YOUR PROGRAMS

There's nothing wrong with you. You weren't born to fail or to struggle with your weight. You don't have some "character flaw" that caused the problem, or is stopping you from winning. The problem is in the programs. Your weight, *right now,* is determined by the programs you already have.

Whatever is in those programs is playing a vital role in your weight and your appearance each day. That means how much you *weigh,* how you *look,* and even much of how you *feel,* is directly affected or determined by the programs you already have. And in order to find out what to *do* about those programs—and the weight problems they cause—let's take a look at how programming actually works.

Chapter Five
The Strongest Program Always Wins

Why is it that one person can easily push away a half-finished plate of food without even thinking about it—while another person will eat everything that's there and still want more? Why do most diet programs, that seem to work for a while, eventually *stop* working?

When I first began looking into the problems of weight control, I asked myself those questions and many others.

Is the problem with weight more physical or more mental?

Why do some people crave sweets and fat, while other people don't?

Why do we feel the need to eat everything on our plate?

Is there really a physical "time clock" that makes weight gain inevitable?

How is it that two people from the same family can be so different weight-wise?

What makes us overeat?

Why is losing weight (or keeping it off) easy for some people and difficult for others?

Why do people lose weight and then gain back more than they lost?

Why do even the so-called "good" diet programs eventually fail for most of the people who try them?

What really causes most weight problems in the first place?

The answer to each of those questions lies in a recent discovery that has to do with the chemical makeup and activity of the human brain.

We have discovered that when people understand what the *problem* really is, they often do a much better job of getting in control of their weight and staying in control. Just *understanding* how the process works can't solve the weight problem by *itself*, but it can offer you tremendous help.

YOUR PROGRAMS REALLY EXIST—THEY ARE ACTUAL *PATHWAYS* IN THE BRAIN

Your programs are real. They are actually patterns of neurons that are physically linked together—like chemical, neurological highways—*"pathways" in your brain*.

All of the messages you got were recorded in those program paths. Everything you did. Everything you said. Everything you heard, experienced, or even thought. And with every repeated use, those neuron pathways got stronger and stronger. The more you used them, the more you traveled over the same highways in your brain, the more you "fed" them—that is, the more chemical nutrition you gave them, and the stronger they got.

And *everything* you think or do today is a result of those programs.

Every time you *do* the same thing, *think* the same thing, *hear* the same message, or *say* the same message, you are walking over the same neuron paths in your brain, again and again. Each time you do, you're actually *feeding* the neurons in those pathways—you're giving them chemical nutrients, so *those* pathways get stronger. In time, the paths you use most become the highways and the super-highways.

Each time, as an example, we looked in the mirror and told ourself this diet wouldn't work, we gave more chemical strength to *that* program in our brain. Each time we took the extra bite, cleaned the plate when we shouldn't have, told ourselves we'd do something about our weight *next* week, or ate the wrong foods or overate "just this once," we made those programs stronger and stronger.

And in time, one by one, each of the programs were formed into chemical patterns, *cemented* into place in our brains and in our lives.

THE RETURN OF THE "HOT 100"

In an earlier book, I included a list of 100 of the most typically "negative" self-talk phrases I had collected from people over the years. I call the list my "Hot 100." In reviewing this list, note how many of the seemingly "harmless" self-talk phrases it contains apply directly to weight problems, or indicate deeper programs that reflect attitudes and habits which tie in with not being fully in control of our lives. In reality, none of these self-talk phrases is *harmless* at all.

As you read through this list of *negative* self-talk, see if you know someone who says something similar, or if you have said something like any of these yourself:

I can't remember names.
It's going to be another one of those days!
It's just no use!
I just know it won't work!
Nothing ever goes right for me.
That's just my luck.
I'm so clumsy.
I don't have the talent.
I'm just not creative.
Everything I eat goes right to my waist.
I can't seem to get organized.
Today just isn't my day!
I can never afford the things I want.
I already know I won't like it.
No matter what I do, I can't seem to lose weight.
I never have enough time.
I just don't have the patience for that.
That really makes me mad!
Another blue Monday!
When will I ever learn!
I get sick just thinking about it.
Sometimes I just hate myself.
I'm just no good!
I'm too shy.
I never know what to say.
With my luck I don't have a chance!
I'd like to stop smoking but I can't seem to quit.

Things just aren't working out right for me.
I don't have the energy I used to.
I'm really out of shape.
I never have any money left over at the end of the month.
Why should I try—it's not going to work anyway!
I've never been any good at that.
My desk is always a mess!
The only kind of luck I have is bad luck!
I never win anything!
I feel like I'm over the hill.
Someone always beats me to it!
Nobody likes me.
I never get a break!
It seems like I'm always broke!
Everything I touch turns to "bleep."
Nobody wants to pay me what I'm worth.
Sometimes I wish I'd never been born!
I'm just no good at math.
I lose weight, but then I gain it right back again.
I get so depressed!
I just can't seem to get anything done!
Nothing seems to go right for me!
I'm just not a salesperson.
That's impossible!
There's just no way!
I always freeze up in front of a group.
I'm nothing without my first cup of coffee in the morning.
I just can't get with it today.
I'll never get it right!
I just can't take it anymore!
I hate my job.
I get a cold this time every year.
I'm really at the end of my rope.
You can't trust anyone anymore!
I just can't handle this!

I never seem to get anyplace on time.
I've always been bad with words.
If only I were smarter.
If only I were taller.
If only I had more time.
If only I had more money.
If only I were thinner ...
... and on, and on, and on.

And those kinds of programs are just a brief glimpse of the deeper programs that lie below! Imagine sitting down at your personal computer keyboard and typing any one of those directions into the computer, knowing what we now know about how our self-talk actually gets programmed *physically* in our brains!

And now imagine that your computer will do whatever you program it to do—because *it will.*

It's no *wonder* that we fail to get where we are trying to go in our lives when we take a look at some of the strong programs we've been living with.

The rule is:

The strongest program always wins.

That means that when any question comes up that has to do with your weight, like "Do I eat this, or don't I?" what you do next will be the result of the programs you have that are strongest.

Let's take a look at some of the specific programs we have right now about *dieting, exercise,* and *eating.*

Chapter Six

Programs About Dieting, Exercise, And Eating

Some of our worst programs come from the very process of dieting and exercise that was supposed to solve our weight problems in the first place. Why do so many people gain weight just before they are about to go on a diet—or gain the weight back when the diet stops? It is because diets *themselves* give us programs that cause us to be dissatisfied, teach us to not believe in ourselves, lower our self-esteem, and eventually, create *more* of the problem and more of the weight.

"DIETING" CREATES PROGRAMS THAT WORK *AGAINST* YOU

As Dr. Schwartz tells us, "Diets are supposed to make us think less about food, but just the reverse happens. *Anything human beings are deprived of, they become obsessive about.* When we think of dieting, we begin to think about food all the time. We even have *dreams* about eating!"

Dr. Schwartz is right. Think about the internal messages most people receive from dieting, or even *thinking* about dieting.

SOME OF OUR OLD PROGRAMS
ABOUT DIETING

"If I don't stay on this diet, I'll gain weight."

"It's hard for me to eat the right kind of food."

"I'd rather be eating something I like."

"I hate diets."

"I'll never lose weight!"

"Food that's good for me doesn't taste good."

"No diet ever works for me."

"I lose the weight but then I gain it right back again."

"It's hopeless!"

"No matter how hard I try, it never works for me!"

"When I stop the diet, the weight will come back."

"It might work for a while but then it will quit."

"Other people can do it but I can't."

"Why should I even try?"

"It's too much work for what I get out of it."

"It's not worth it."

"There must be something wrong with me because I have to diet."

"Going on a diet makes me gain weight."

"I'll always be overweight!"

"Diets are expensive."

"Diet food always tastes bad."

"Diets are depressing."

"I'll always be on a diet!"

All of those internal messages and dozens of other messages just like them are actually programs. Every time we hear them, say them, think them, or when they cross our mind unconsciously, *one more program is being recorded, chemically and electrically in our subconscious mind.* One more program is being *added* to the other negative "diet" programs already working against us.

OUR OLD PROGRAMS ABOUT EXERCISING

We all know that the right kind of exercise is good for us. In his health clubs, Dr. Schwartz saw the first-hand results of proper exercise in thousands of people's lives. According to Dr. Schwartz—along with many other experts in his field—the benefits exercise can bring are many and varied:

1. Exercise is an effective way to rid yourself of stress and can prevent overeating caused by stress.

2. Exercise releases pent-up energy and frustration.

3. Exercise causes almost immediate improvement in the way you look. Exercise tightens and tones loose, flabby muscles. Losing inches becomes the motivation to exercise even more.

4. Exercising allows you to use time, once spent over-eating, in a productive and fun way.

5. Exercising is a great way to meet and receive the support of other people who are also motivated to be physically fit, feel their best, and lead healthy lives.

However, even Dr. Schwartz himself cautions against the belief that exercise alone will make you lose weight. He says, "The purpose of exercise is to be physically fit, to feel and look your best. You can be physically fit and still be overweight.

"It takes *thirty minutes* of aerobic dancing to burn off twelve corn chips. Does it take anyone you know thirty minutes to eat twelve corn chips? Probably not. The bottom line is that the fastest exerciser cannot burn up the number of calories that even the slowest overeater can take in."

So as Dr. Schwartz points out, most of us have unrealistic or mistaken expectations—and erroneous *programs*—when it comes to the value of exercise for losing weight. Here is an example of the kinds of programs many people have learned to give themselves every time they exercise, or even *think* about exercising:

"I'm too lazy."

"I hate to exercise."

"The more I exercise the more weight I gain."

"I never have enough time to exercise."

"I'm too tired."

"I get started but I never stick to it."

"I've started a million exercise programs."

"The more I exercise, the more I want to eat."

"Exercising just makes me think about food!"

"I can get started, but I can't stay with it."

"This exercise machine will probably end up in the garage with all the others."

"I hurt when I exercise."

"It's not worth the effort it takes."

The same is true of weight-loss programs that focus too heavily on *eating* or on *eating habits*. Neurologically, like the "diet" and the "exercise" messages we just looked at, every time we focus on "eating," we add another batch of negative programs to our already-crowded program files on wanting to eat. In so doing we add more support to the other programs we already have *that are just like them*.

OUR OLD PROGRAMS ABOUT EATING

"Just thinking about trying to lose weight makes me want to eat."

"I just love to eat!"

"I'm afraid I won't be able to eat the things I like."

"Anything that tastes good is bad for me."

"It's too complicated to eat the right food."

"Just look at all those good things I wish I could eat!"

"Just this once won't hurt."

"I'll just have one more bite."

"I eat when I'm bored."

"I eat when I get depressed."

"I eat when I'm lonely."

"I eat when I'm feeling good."

"Everything I eat goes right to my thighs."

"All I ever think about is eating!"

(If your programs about eating sound anything like these, I recommend you try Dr. Schwartz's "naturally thin" technique, "A Taste Of The Thin Life," in Part III .)

WHAT ARE THE PROGRAMS *YOUR* "COMPUTER" IS FOLLOWING?

Are all of your programs the *right* programs, or would you like to trade some of them in for a few *different* ones? That's an important question, because your programs don't stop with their effect on your weight. They influence *everything in your life.*

Everything you do about dieting, exercise, and eat-ing—*or anything else in your life*—is determined by the strongest programs you have cemented in place right now in your brain.

Let's take a look at the programs *you* have that could be controlling your weight—and a whole lot more.

Chapter Seven
Seven Programs That Control Your Weight

Wouldn't it be interesting to walk up to a special computer printer and plug it directly into your subconscious mind, push the "print" button, and print out all of the tens of thousands of programs that are locked up inside your brain?

LOOKING INTO "THE FILING CABINETS" OF YOUR MIND

Let's say you would like to take a look at your own programs. In order to do that, let's take a walk upstairs into your computer center and take a look around. We'll go on a guided tour, like a NASA tour, and I'll be your tour guide. We will begin by imagining that the two of us are standing in the middle of a large warehouse room.

In the front of the room is a giant computer screen. That's where all of your computer's directions to you are typed out. The walls of the room are covered, floor to ceiling, with *thousands* of filing cabinets. Each of these filing cabinets is filled to overflowing with file folders,

41

and those file folders contain *all of the programs you've ever received.*

Looking around, we see that the filing cabinets are separated into sections. They include the seven primary program files that control your weight.

These seven primary program sections include:

1. *Health and Physical Fitness*
2. *Personal Responsibility*
3. *Personal Motivation*
4. *Self-Esteem*
5. *Deserving to Succeed*
6. *Habits and Actions*
7. *Programs of Success and Failure*

Now, as we walk around the room, we are surrounded by all those program files. We can, if we choose, look into any of them and find out what's inside. To get an idea of what's in them, we'll look into just a few.

SEVEN PRIMARY "PROGRAM FILES" THAT CONTROL YOUR WEIGHT

1. Programs About Your "Health and Physical Fitness"

In this section of files, we find your programs on *Personal Appearance, Physical Health, Diet, Exercise, Nutrition, Food, Eating Habits. . .* and as we suspected, this is the section of files where all of your programs about *Weight-Loss* are stored. You could look into these files and find everything you *know*, or *believe*, or have *ever experienced* about weight-loss and diets and dieting, and

42

every related program.

Let us say you decided to set a goal to lose weight. Typically, you would then set the amount of weight you wanted to lose, and decide how long it would take. You might, if you're serious enough, write down the goal. If you're especially dedicated, you might even draw a graph to plot your results over a period of weeks or months.

Let us also say that this goal is important to you. Not only is it important to lose the weight itself, but it is equally important to prove to yourself once and for all that you can do it! You deserve to take the weight off and to get in shape—and stay that way. So the goal you set is not just a whim. It's a serious goal. Reaching it will have a positive effect on your relationships, your work, and in other areas of your life.

If, at the point you set the goal, you already know something about programming, you might decide to work on some of your old "overweight" programs. So you decide to change what you eat, how much you eat, when and where you eat, and anything else that could help you reach the goal you have set. You try to work on the programs you have that are filed under the program sections titled *"Weight-Loss"* and *"Diets & Dieting."*

But if one of the neuroscientists who studies neuron paths in the brain were there to coach you, I suspect she or he might tell you that dealing with *those* programs— the programs that deal directly with food and dieting— might be *exactly* the wrong programs to work on!

If you wanted to find the programs that are causing the weight problem, I suspect the neuroscientist would have you look at the sets of files in a *different* section altogether. As an example, you might want to look into the next section of programs. This section is filled with program files that determine how much responsibility you take for yourself and for every action you take—

about anything—every moment:

2. Programs About Your "Personal Responsibility"

The programs that fill this section can be any programs that have allowed you to give up taking responsibility for yourself or for any part of your life, no matter how minor.

Some people go through their entire lives letting other people do their breathing for them. When you think about it, once we reach adulthood, it doesn't make any sense to let someone *else* live or direct part of *our* lives *for* us. And, yet, it happens to many people all the time. Perhaps no one has ever said anything like the following to you, but I have heard each of these comments spoken by otherwise caring individuals, to someone they loved:

"Honey, why even try? You know you're never going to lose any weight." "You don't need to lose an ounce!" "You don't need to change...I like you better just the way you are!" "Go ahead, one piece of cake isn't going to hurt you." "I don't want you to go on another one of your silly diets." "I can just see you...first you lose the weight, and the next thing you know, you'll want to go back to work and never be home."

Those examples are clearly pointed at weight. But what about the *other* pushes and tugs and manipulations that are far less obvious; but may be far more controlling in our lives?

I met one woman at a seminar who told me she is still trying to live up to the expectations of her father. The problem, she finally concluded, was that she has never been able to please her father, even though she has tried for years to live the way *he* would prefer she lives. And she also correctly concluded that because her father always disapproved of her when she looked slim and sexy, no matter *what* weight program she went on, the moment she got looking "good" again—read as, "too sexy"—back would come the weight.

She was still trying to live so her father would approve of her. She had given up her own personal responsibility for herself to programs that were stronger than she was—and they were in control. She was still trying to live up to the programs her father had created.

Those were powerful programs, and they would not let her go. That was unfortunate. The woman I was talking to was fifty-eight. Her father had been dead for thirty-seven years.

3. *Programs About Your "Personal Motivation"*

There is another set of programs that is always found near the heart of how well you will succeed at dealing with weight. These are the programs that control your *motivation*.

In this section of your program files are all of the programs you have that either put you in motion, or hold you back. In this section you will find the programs that have caused you to procrastinate, or put off doing things that were good for you, things you had intended to do.

If you have *any* programs of *"Personal Motivation"* that tell you it's okay to *put it off* or delay, those programs will not go away just because you set a new goal or tell yourself it is going to be different this time.

If, in the past, you ever wondered why you avoided doing what you knew you *should*, we could learn from reading through the programs in these files, *exactly* what stopped you in the first place.

If you looked closely, what do you suppose you would find in *your* files on "motivation" right now?

4. Programs About Your "Self-Esteem"

A very large section of your computer control center is filled with the programs that make up your "Self-Esteem."

It is *here*, in these important files, that we would find the programs that have shaped all of your opinions and attitudes and beliefs about yourself.

It is here that you will find the programs that tell you who you are, the programs that shape your character, your will, your determination, and the complete, composite picture of who you believe yourself to be.

If you have self-esteem programs that tell you that slim, trim, attractive person is not *you*, then in spite of how hard you try, the person in the mirror will eventually be like the person whose picture is stored in those programs.

How is your self-esteem right now? What kind of programs do you have about yourself? What do you *really* believe about who you are and what you *can* do? Is there anything that is holding you back? What do your self-esteem programs *really* tell you?

If you want to lose weight, to get in control, you will find an important part of your answer here, in the program files that make up your *self-esteem*.

5. Programs About Your "Deserving to Succeed"

Close to your program files of self-esteem, you will find a section of programs called "Deserving To Succeed."

Do you have *any* programs that tell you that you belong in second place, or third, or that you come in last, or not at all? Do you have any programs that tell you *others* come first, or that you simply were not designed to succeed in the first place? If you have *any* programs that tell you—no matter how subtly—that you do not *deserve* to succeed, then no matter how hard you try, no matter how many diets you start, no matter how often you reach the top for a time—those old programs will step back in, and take over once again. They will pull you back to the place in your life *where they believe you belong*.

6. Programs About Your "Habits and Actions"

All of our habits and actions are governed by our programs. But in time, our strongest habits and our most consistent actions get filed in their own special section. We can even notice it happening when it happens to us. We will say something we shouldn't have said, and then hear ourself saying, "Now why did I say that? I know better than that!" Or we will pick up the fork, and reach for another bite of cake, without even noticing what we have done. It is an action—now a program—that by now is so strong that it has a life of its own.

We can promise ourselves we will not yell at the kids anymore, and then that night, yell at them louder than before. We can resolutely tell ourselves that we will save the money and not spend it for anything, no matter how much we want it—and then watch in almost hypnotic amazement as we buy something because it was on sale.

"Habits" are not just those behaviors we think of as "bad" habits or "good." *Habits make up anything we do without having to think about it.* And all of our habits are made up of program paths in the brain.

If you want to get in control of your weight, but you have *any* habits or actions that have worked against you in the past, those same programs will be there just as strong tomorrow. Those programs filed in your program section labeled *"Habits and Actions,"* whatever they are, will not stop being there just because you *want* to make a change. The same habits and repeated actions that got you through last week will be with you next week as well.

What are the "habit" programs you have right now? Do you have any habits that get in your way? Do you have any patterns of behavior that make you gain weight or keep it on, when a different habit would be better for you?

Habits are programs. If you find any here that have stopped you in the past, those are programs that will try just as hard to stop you in the future.

7. Programs About Your "Success and Failure"

There is another section of files that get filled up as time goes by, and eventually these programs become some of our strongest programs of all. These files are made up of thousands of moments of minor successes and failures—most of them forgotten. In time those successes and failures form a pathway of expectations and beliefs about your ability to succeed.

We measure each new endeavor against the successes and failures that preceded it. It is our success or failure programs that unconsciously cast the vote in advance; we *predict* our own futures based on the *"Success and Failure"* programs from our past. Unfortunately, these are strong programs, programs that may *tell* us we are going to *fail*, even if we could have succeeded.

But we follow the path of unconscious self-suggestions and are led to the failure that we so accurately predicted. Even the simple comments, *"I just know I'll never lose this weight,"* or *"It's just no use,"* not only show the powerful programs that are hidden behind the thoughts, but even in saying the words, we help create the failure before we have even gotten started.

What are the success or failure programs you carry with you right now? When you're thinking of losing weight or keeping it off, what do you find in your program files that tell you how well you're going to do this time?

Whatever is there, *those* are the programs that *want* to stay in control.

THERE ARE MANY MORE PROGRAMS THAT CAN AFFECT YOUR WEIGHT

Many other programs can affect your goal to lose weight or keep it off. These could have to do with any other aspect of your life. A few of these include your programs of *Personal Relationships; Money; Talents and Ability; Honesty; Attitudes* of every kind; how you deal with *Stress;* programs of *Recognition* and *Approval; Security and Insecurity; Determination and Willpower;* and many others.

The files we've just looked at are only a few examples of the thousands you have stored right now in your computer control center, and each of these programs can in some way affect whether you will or will not reach your goal, and get in control of your weight.

The important thing to remember is that many of the programs that cause our weight problems don't have to have anything to do with weight—at least not on the surface.

A WOMAN NAMED LISA

I knew a woman named Lisa who would lose weight, almost reach her goal, and then, very rapidly, gain it all back again. Over a period of time I watched Lisa do this time and time again. I also noticed that each time Lisa lost the weight, she would start to get very pretty again. Her weight swings would take her from overweight and unhealthy, to trim and very attractive.

After observing Lisa following this same pattern repeatedly, I decided to observe her behavior more closely, to see if I could discover what was behind her gain/loss/gain cycle.

At this particular time, Lisa's self-esteem was the lowest she could ever remember—and it had always been very low. She weighed more now than ever. None of her clothes fit, not even the largest sizes. Nothing she could do would hide the weight anymore, not even from herself. Looking in the mirror made her shake her head; she would look away to avoid what she saw. It got to the point where Lisa wouldn't go out socially at all. She found it too depressing.

Lisa decided once again that she would have to get herself under control. Somehow, in the midst of her unhappiness, she decided to try one more time.

And so, once again Lisa followed her old programs, and started the pattern over. Her next "diet" was the starvation kind—temporary and unhealthy. Lisa had done it many times before, only *this time* she was determined that it would be different. This time she would not only reach her goal, she would *keep* the weight off—or so she thought.

Lisa's friends began to notice the difference by the

second or third week, and her attitude began to improve as the pounds came off. In six weeks people were starting to make complimentary remarks about how good she looked. After eight weeks one of her associates, a single man from work, asked her to go out with him. She didn't go, but two or three weeks after that another man, a casual friend who was married, began to hint around at the two of them getting together sometime.

Day by day Lisa was becoming more attractive again— she was naturally pretty, and without the weight to hide her attractive appearance, people started to notice her "differently." Just when Lisa was finally about to reach her weight-loss goal, she suddenly realized that people were placing new expectations on her—and although it seemed that everyone was joining in with new expectations, it was the men who seemed to expect the most.

The more attractive she became, the more uncomfortable she got. And it was then that Lisa began to feel things were starting to close in on her. People were getting too expecting, too demanding, too intimate, too *close*.

What do you suppose Lisa did next? She did the only thing she knew to do—the one thing she had always done before. And the one thing she could do that was guaranteed to push the world away was *eat*.

Within a few short weeks, not only had Lisa put all of the weight back on, faster than she had taken it off in the first place, but she'd added a few *more* pounds for good measure. And sure enough, the new demands on her went away.

There is no greater blanket of security between us and the rest of the world than the security of weight, safely walling us off from the uncaring world around us, and keeping that world at bay. Once again, *Lisa was safe*. And she blamed her failure to lose the weight, on the latest *diet* she had been on!

It was *exactly* what Lisa had done before—and if nothing happened to change her pattern, it was *exactly* what she would do again.

WHAT WERE THE PROGRAMS THAT CAUSED LISA TO FAIL?

Where would you look for the programs that had once again caused Lisa to fail?

If we could walk upstairs into Lisa's computer storage center, I would not look in the section of program files marked *"Diets"* or *"Weight-Loss"* for the programs that were causing her to fail. The programs that caused Lisa's problem with weight, as with so many of us, had little or nothing to do with her "weight-loss" programs. Weight is almost always a symptom of *other* things going on in our lives.

If we wanted to help Lisa find the real programs that were causing her problem, I would first look into those program files marked *"Security and Insecurity."* I would then look at the programs in the section headed *"Personal Relationships."* I would be sure to look at the programs called *"Self-Esteem."* I would look for the faulty programs in the diet and weight-loss section *last*—if at *all*.

And if we wanted to help Lisa end her weight-loss battle for good—and *win*—I would show her how to get her old programs to stop voting *against* her and get them to start voting in her favor.

Chapter Eight
Who's Voting On Your Weight?

Imagine that we are standing right now in the middle of your computer control center with its thousands of filing cabinets, and one by one we read over the titles on each of the sections:

Health and Physical Fitness
Personal Responsibility
Personal Motivation
Self-Esteem
Deserving to Succeed
Habits and Actions
Success and Failure
Personal Relationships
Money and Financial Freedom
Dealing With Stress
Honesty
Recognition and Approval
Talents and Ability
Security and Insecurity
Determination and Will Power
and so on . . .

Now imagine you could walk up to any one of those filing cabinets, in any of the sections, and open it up and look inside.

What do you suppose you would find in your files? In those files you would find your dreams, your hopes, your failings and your fears. In them you would find your strengths and your hesitations, your goals and your uncertainties, and the most complete picture ever found of who you are today, and who you *could* be tomorrow.

And in those files you would find every one of your beliefs—and the script that is even *now* being written for the future that is yet in front of you.

YOUR PROGRAMS TAKE A VOTE—
THEIR VOTE DECIDES YOUR WEIGHT

The effect of our programs on our day-to-day actions is far stronger than we ever knew. In the past, when we have even thought the words *"weight-loss,"* or *"diet,"* we've automatically opened the program files in our brain that had anything to do with the subject of weight. Some of the programs we carried were good programs, and some were bad—negative programs, or programs that led us in unhealthy directions.

But even more apparent is that it wasn't our programs about *weight* itself that were the real culprits; it was the *other* programs we carried—programs that on the surface seemed to have nothing to do with weight at all.

Even when we *think* we're thinking about weight itself, our brain is silently sorting through those *other* files that are actually the *cause* of most of our failure. The moment the word "diet" even enters our mind, dozens of other filing cabinets open up, at lightning speed, and hundreds of individual program files come flying out.

And in that same instant, those programs take a *vote.*

Every thought, every action is voted on by every single program file in your brain that could have anything at all to do with what you will do or think next. To show you how this voting process works, let's look at a real-life example.

A NEW DIET FOR DORIS

A woman I met, named Doris, told me she had fought a losing battle with weight for many years. She would lose weight, but then something would happen and she would stop short of her goal. Doris was good at dieting. In fact, she had tried them all. She would stay with each one for a while, and then fall off. Her weight went from moderate to heavy to slim to heavy again, time after time.

Finally Doris decided this was it! She was *through* half-doing it. *This* time she was going to stay with it. So she found yet another diet plan and got started. She set her goal, wrote it down, took her measurements, wrote them down, stepped on the scale, wrote her weight down, and then stepped forward to meet the new life that she hoped was in front of her.

This time what she was doing appeared to work better than it had in the past. She watched what she ate, exercised, and the pounds began to come off. In a short time everyone else was noticing it too. And even though it was a struggle, after months of hard work she was finally within ten pounds of her ultimate goal.

Then one Wednesday, Doris was invited to go to lunch with a group of women from her office. She knew she still had ten pounds to go, so at lunch Doris ordered a salad with a low-calorie, low-fat Caesar dressing, and waved away the rolls and the margarine that went with it. She ordered tea to drink, and then, proud of herself, she engaged in an intense discussion with two of her friends seated across from her.

After the entrees were finished, while Doris was still in the middle of her discussion with her friends, the waiter came to their table with the dessert tray. On the tray, right in front, was something called "Death by Chocolate." Doris stopped talking for a moment and looked longingly at the dessert, and then in a forced surge of resolve, she shook her head "no," and turned back to her friends.

As Doris and the friends continued their talk, completely immersed in the conversation, another "friend," seated two seats away at the table, ordered the chocolate cake *for* Doris, and then quietly slid it toward her across the table. (Obviously, this person was *not* a real friend.)

Without her even noticing it, and while she continued to talk, Doris's right hand slowly picked up her dessert fork, and then her hand with the fork in it just as slowly moved toward the chocolate cake that had been so unkindly placed in front of her. Finally, still talking intently to her friends, and without even thinking about it, Doris raised her fork above the dessert.

WATCH WHAT'S REALLY HAPPENING

At that moment, "freeze-frame" Doris! Stop her right there with her dessert fork poised in mid-air, ready to attack the cake and sabotage the diet, or return to the table and boost her success.

Now, rush upstairs into Doris's computer control center

and watch what's really happening at that precise moment! In that instant, Doris's computer filing cabinets
begin flying open at lightning speed! In that same
moment, every program in Doris's entire program storage center that has *anything at all* to do with what Doris
will do next, will *vote*. In that instant, all of those programs fly out—and each one votes—with the *stronger*
programs always out-voting the *weaker* programs.

Doris's programs on how well she has done in the past;
her programs that tell her how good she is at setting
goals and reaching them; her programs that create her
security and insecurity; programs that tell her whether
she accepts responsibility for every action she takes; her
programs of personal motivation, procrastination, and
getting things done; programs from her recent past and
programs from long ago; all of her programs of *self-esteem*—who she really is, how much self-worth she has,
and everything she believes about herself—in that same
moment, all of those programs—and thousands more just
like them—*vote!*

And *in that same moment* the vote is tallied up, and the
results instantly type themselves across the giant computer screen in Doris's computer control center.

Whatever is written on that screen will determine what
Doris will do next. Every program has voted, chemically
and electrically, biologically, *neurologically* in her
brain—all in a single *instant* of time!

At that moment, on the computer control screen in
Doris's internal control center, the words read:

"*Okay to eat one bite.*"

Now take Doris out of freeze-frame. In less than the
space of a single heartbeat, the decision has been made.
Doris's fork continues toward the chocolate cake . . . *and*

she takes the bite.

During the next few minutes that same scenario will be repeated six or seven times—until there is no more "Death by Chocolate" left on the plate in front of her. It also signals the "death" of her diet.

There is no doubt that Doris, in that moment, made a bad decision. It was a decision that would prove to hurt her. In fact, in real life, within a week of that incident, Doris had stopped her diet completely. She not only failed to reach her goal, but she began gaining the weight back again—faster this time than she had lost it in the first place. Her self-esteem plummeted. She had gotten *so close*. Success had been almost in her grasp.

Later, through the haze of depression she fell into, Doris once again blamed the diet. She said it was another diet that could not live up to its claims. And she blamed herself. She had gone to lunch, blown her diet, beaten up on herself, and within days, had failed completely. That moment at lunch was just the first step.

I would agree that Doris made a bad choice at lunch that day. Despite the unkindness her so-called friend had shown her by ordering the cake for Doris, it was still up to Doris to make the right decision for herself.

But something else is going on here. More important forces were at play than a noon lunch, a forbidden dessert, and a bad decision.

WHAT *REALLY* MADE THE CHOICE FOR DORIS?

The truth is that *Doris did not really make a conscious choice at all!* At the moment the decision to eat the cake was being made, *Doris was not even thinking about her diet.* She was intently involved in a conversation with her friends across the table. She did not stop and think about it, nor was she aware that a vote was being taken. She did not make a conscious decision herself. She didn't have to. *Doris's internal programs made the decision <u>for</u> her.*

While she was busy thinking about something else, Doris's programs voted, decided, and swung into action. It was *those* programs that wanted Doris to eat. It was her old programs that wanted Doris to stop struggling, and give up and go back to being her *"normal"* overweight self.

It wasn't what Doris consciously *wanted*—it was what her programs were designed to get her to do. Those programs wanted to take Doris back to the *old* way of being. They were *designed* to. In this minor, yet singularly important event in her life, Doris was *programmed* to fail.

It was Doris's programs that did the voting *for* her, just as *our* programs do most of our voting for us. If Doris had different programs—healthier programs of strong positive self-esteem, programs that saw her as deserving and worthwhile, programs of strong self-motivation, and programs that would insure her on-going physical and emotional healthiness—with the *right* kinds of programs, the outcome of Doris's vote would have been far different. And so might her *life* have been different!

What if someone had been able to help Doris change those old programs? What if she could have gotten rid of them, exchanged them for the kind of programs that would help her live up to the life she really *wanted*—and deserved—to live?

It is clear that our programs have a major impact on our lives—and on every single action we take. And unless we do something to *change* those old programs, we will continue to fail. *The old programs will continue to vote against us.*

A BOY NAMED EDDIE

During my in-person seminars, I often meet individuals who share with me the stories of what programming did to their lives. Their stories prove how programming affects *every* area of people's lives—far beyond such things as controlling our weight.

I remember one couple in particular who talked with me after a seminar. I will never forget the story they told me about their young son, Eddie. So often, I have pictured the way it must have happened. A particular day in that young man's life went much like this:

Eddie is sixteen years old. He is on his way to school one Monday morning. As he walks, he is thinking intently about a test he has to take that morning. He's right on time; it's about ten minutes to eight.

Eddie is in the street, about to step up onto the curb and then onto the sidewalk that leads to the front door of the school, when up the street toward him drives a car at high speed. The car comes screeching to a halt less than a foot and a half from where Eddie is walking. The windows of the car are rolled down, and inside are four of Eddie's friends. They yell, *"Hey Eddie—let's cut class!"*

Freeze-frame Eddie right there, with one foot in midair, about to step up onto the sidewalk, ready to either continue on his way to class—or change his path and join his friends.

Now, rush upstairs into Eddie's computer control center and watch as program file after program file flies open at lightning speed, as one by one the programs cast their vote! Every one of Eddie's programs that has *anything at all* to do with what he is going to do next, will *vote*—the stronger programs always out-voting the weaker ones.

Every file that has anything to do with Eddie's education . . .how well he's done in school up until now. . .whether he thinks he's capable or not. . .all of Eddie's files on self-esteem. . .how important it is to go along with the crowd, or not. . .what he believes about the importance of staying in school. . .all of Eddie's programs vote and *in that same instant*, the results are tallied up. And across Eddie's computer control screen scroll the words:

"Okay to cut class."

Un-freeze-frame Eddie. Eddie turns, jumps into the car, and in a spray of dust and gravel, the car speeds away.

Eddie made a bad decision. I would never absolve Eddie of the responsibility he had to make the right choice for himself. And yet, who really made the choice for Eddie? *He wasn't even thinking about it!* He was thinking about the test he had to take that day. At no time do I recall Eddie saying, "Wait a minute, guys. Do any of you have a pencil and a legal pad? I'd like to think through a logical decision on this. I'll draw a line down the middle of the pad, put 'pro' on one side and 'con' on the other, then list 'reasons to stay in school' and 'reasons to cut class. . .'"

No! Eddie didn't have to think about the choice he was asked to make; his old programs made the choice *for* him.

As I said, it was a bad choice. Eddie got punished for cutting class, and he got punished several times after that when he did it again. Eventually, though, he didn't get punished anymore. He stopped going to school entirely, and was no longer living at home. When his parents finally found him, he was in an alley. Eddie didn't even recognize them when they came to take him home because of the drugs and alcohol in his system.

Eddie is a real person. I've met Eddie. I know his parents. Eddie was lucky; his story isn't over yet, because his parents found him in time. But he—and they—have a lot of work to do to repair the damage caused by the wrong programs in Eddie's computer.

Am I convinced that Eddie would have taken a completely different action on the day of that important test, and all the days that followed it, if he'd had different programs on his side? I believe Eddie's story would have been much different if he had different programs to do his voting for him. That's the way our programs work.

There may be no more important single thing we can do in our lives than to make sure that the programs *we* have that do *our* voting for us, are the right programs. If the wrong programs can be strong enough to change someone's path in life, like Eddie's, imagine the effect our programs have on something as simple as controlling what we choose to eat—or *anything* else we do.

DO YOU HAVE ANY PROGRAMS YOU WOULD LIKE TO CHANGE?

Pause for a moment and answer this question for yourself: Are you satisfied with the programs you have right now? Do you have any programs you would like to get rid of? Or, if you could, do you have any programs you would like to change?

We have learned it is the brain that records our programs in the first place, and that brain doesn't care whether those programs are true or false, right or wrong, positive or negative. It simply records them and acts them out. But we have also learned there is a way to get *past* the old programs that have been working against us—and that the brain is designed to *help* us do it. And finally, we have learned *how*.

Chapter Nine

Changing Your Programs— Changing Your Weight

At this point in my research about weight control I reasoned, "It *can't* just stop there; there *has* to be an answer." If programs are actual patterns in the brain, but we could do nothing to *change* any of them, we might have reason to give up. But fortunately, the research led to another *major* breakthrough. The importance of this discovery is so great we are only now beginning to realize what it could mean to each of our lives.

A WAY TO *STOP* THE OLD PROGRAMS

What the researchers discovered can be explained very simply: They learned, while observing neuron pathways in the brain, that if the individual were to *stop* using a program path *long* enough, that neuron pathway would, in time, stop being *fed*, and begin to break down. *It would lose its strength—all by itself!*

What happens to anything organic when you stop feeding it? It gets weaker. It loses its strength and begins to die out. What happens to any program path in the human brain when you stop using it entirely? *It begins to lose its strength and die out.*

IF YOU STOP USING THE OLD PROGRAMS COMPLETELY—THEY BEGIN TO BREAK DOWN!

When you stop traveling on the wrong neuron paths, those chemical highways begin to fall into disuse and disrepair, like a freeway that has been closed and nobody uses anymore. In time the roadway begins to fill with cracks and weeds, gradually breaking down, and eventually becomes unfit for any travel at all.

That illustration describes, in a simplified way, what happens to our program paths in the brain. When we stop giving our brain the same negative or harmful messages, when we stop using those program paths entirely, they begin to break down. They lose their hold over our lives. And it is a *physical* process in the brain!

It was this discovery that told us, for the first time ever, there might be a way to be set free from the old programs that had governed our lives for so long. The old programs *would* lose their strength—*if* somehow we could stop using them long enough for them to begin to break down!

YOU HAVE TO STAY WITH IT LONG ENOUGH FOR IT TO WORK

Meanwhile, the researchers learned that the process

does not happen overnight. Old neuron paths in the brain do not break down just because we stop using them for a few hours or a day or several days or even a week or two. This is what they learned:

The process of breaking down our old programs does not even begin to take place until we have stopped using the old programs for at least three weeks or longer!

We have all heard the old expression, "How long does it take to change a habit?" The answer is, of course, "Twenty-one days." We didn't know it at the time, but the reason is *chemical*. It takes a minimum of about three weeks—*or more*—before the old programs get weak enough to begin to fade. And that is three weeks before the breakdown process even *starts!*

Finally, we have learned why just *wanting* to change, or just putting forth a temporary effort, doesn't work.

It is no wonder, then, that we cannot change our programs just by reading a book, or by making a New Year's resolution, or even by setting a new goal. You have to give the process time to get started. Neuron pathways in the brain do not break down in a few hours. They do not suddenly stop *being* just because we set a goal or tell ourselves we're going to lose weight and keep it off. *That's not how the brain works!*

WE'VE BEEN TRYING TO LOSE WEIGHT THE WRONG WAY

We have been trying to solve the problem the wrong way. We have been working *harder*, thinking that diets and hard work and effort would be rewarded with a slimmer physique. We believed that if we set strong goals, those goals would somehow transform themselves into a better figure. We have spent hours doing exercises that often made our weight problem worse, thinking that because we put forth the effort and exercise we would be rewarded with a trimmer shape and it would stay that way.

We knew better, of course. Deep down inside there was that voice that kept saying, "You've got to be kidding. You know this isn't going to work; this isn't going to last." That wasn't just negative self-talk (which does not help, either). That "still, small voice" we were hearing was the voice of our own programs—programs we carried, hidden deep within our minds, and carried into our lives with every thought and in every action we took.

YOU CAN'T CHANGE PROGRAMS JUST BY *"WANTING"* THEM TO GO AWAY

You cannot get rid of neuron pathways just by telling yourself to change, or by following most self-help techniques. Motivational as they might be, they don't change the physical pathways that make up the actual programs in your brain.

There has never been a single book written that can, by the reading of it, suddenly change the chemical and electrical pathways in the human brain. There has never been a lecture that, simply by listening to it, changed a single neurological pattern in the brain. There has never been a single goal that could, just by the setting of it, change the programs in a person's biochemical computer.

Yet, we read books looking for help. We look for inspiration from motivational talks. We follow complicated self-improvement methods that are supposed to change our lives. We listen to counseling and advice, hoping to find the cure. We set goals and write them down and work hard to follow them, thinking that we have found the answer—if we can just stay with it.

And meanwhile, our old programs have been smiling to themselves and saying, "That's all right. You go ahead and try as hard as you can. But when you get tired, when the bloom of your new devotion fades away, I will be here waiting for you to come back home to me. I will be waiting for you just like before. I will never leave you. *I am your programs.*"

"DIETS" MAKE BAD PROGRAMS *WORSE*

We had it all *backwards.* Instead of getting *off* the old programs, instead of *stopping* using them, we did the opposite. By "focusing" on the diet itself, we focused on the *old* programs *more*, and made them *stronger!* We drove over and over the same neuron highways again and again.

We focused on our weight. We studied our objective. We fought food and struggled with deprivation and hunger. We forced ourselves to follow a painful or boring or seemingly endless regimen of exercises, all the time focusing our minds stronger and stronger on losing the weight. *In doing that, we forced ourselves to go over and over the exact same programs in our brains that we should have gotten off entirely!*

Every time you get the same message—you use the same pathway. Every time you use the same pathway—it gets *stronger*. The result is:

Most diets strengthen the exact program paths that caused the problem in the first place.

So do most exercise programs. So do most *all* weight-loss techniques we have ever tried. It is no wonder they fail; *they cause us to reinforce the old programs that were working against us in the first place.*

All you have to do is *think* about food—in the *old* way—and you open up the precise filing cabinets in your brain that you should be closing for good. Every time you work at exercising—in the old way—you pull open every filing cabinet in your brain that has anything at all to do with fatigue, hard work, exertion, and failure. And you make those files stronger. When we have been working—*in the old way*—at removing *pounds*, we have, instead, been adding *programs*.

FINALLY, THERE'S HOPE

The real breakthrough is that we *can* get past our old programs. There is a *natural* process that will help us do just that. But we weren't born with an instruction manual for our brains, and it has taken us the entire history of humankind to find out what to do. Imagine trying to program a complicated computer at the office without any reference manuals. You'd give up before you started; it would be impossible. And yet, that's exactly what we've been doing every day, in our own lives, with our own mental computers.

The mistake we have been making is that we tried to get rid of our old programs by focusing on them. We now know that is the opposite of what we should have been doing:

To get rid of an old program, you first have to replace it with something else.

If you want to stop using the old pathways in your brain, you need a new set of pathways to use in their place. And now, for the first time, we have discovered how to create those *new* program paths so that we get where we want to go—instead of where our *old* programs have been trying to send us.

Chapter Ten

The Most *"Natural"* Solution We've Found

We have learned that the old program pathways will break down *only* if we stop using them. It was only recently, of course, that we learned that all this happened chemically and electrically in the brain. But even before that, we had suspected that to make any real changes in our lives we had to somehow magically stop *thinking* like we used to think. That was an early and somewhat naive approach to the problem, but it was looking in the right direction.

The old belief among "self-improvement" enthusiasts was that if we just worked at changing what we think or what we like, we could then, logically, change what we *do* about anything. But that belief did not take into account the fact that *everything* we think and do is the result of the programs that are hidden within us. To truly change what we think, we first have to change the *programs* that created our thoughts in the first place.

The most "natural" and most effective solution we have ever found for controlling your weight long-term is by applying the concept now known as "Self-Talk." That is because the process called Self-Talk is the most natural way we've ever found to get rid of old programs in the brain, and *replace* them with *new programs*—this time, programs of your own choice. And as many medical doctors, therapists and counselors attest, Self-Talk is not only a proven tool, it is something that should be taught to all of us.

CHANGING YOUR PROGRAMS—*AND YOUR WEIGHT*—WITH SELF-TALK

Self-Talk is a method—or rather, a *group* of methods and techniques—that when used together, follow the natural programming processes of the human brain. Because the techniques are designed to work *the way the brain was designed to work in the first place*, Self-Talk is natural. It can be used by anyone who wants to improve his or her programs.

Even children in grade school are learning to use Self-Talk techniques. Self-Talk is easy enough for anyone at any age to use. In Part II of this book, in the section entitled *Self-Talk Techniques*, there are specific steps that are outlined for you to follow.

The purpose is to create the *right* kind of internal programs that will help you get in control of your weight—and *stay* in control of it permanently. Used correctly, Self-Talk will help you do that. But it will also help you *un*consciously. That is, Self-Talk is designed to work for you even while you're not thinking about it or working *at* it.

Because Self-Talk deals with the human brain, and with the programs that determine our thoughts, beliefs, attitudes, and actions, some people might think that Self-Talk is a "new age" concept or a new method of "self- therapy." Nothing could be further from the truth.

WHAT SELF-TALK IS NOT

Self-Talk is not "new age." It is not some new form of self-therapy. It is neither hypnosis nor is it "subliminal." It is not occult, nor does it have *anything* to do with mysticism, or any form of mind control. Self-Talk is the *opposite* of any of these. Instead of turning your programs (and therefore your mind) over to someone else, or some outside force or agency, Self-Talk turns control of your *choices* back over to *you*.

Years ago, when little was understood about Self-Talk, I was asked on a television interview if Self-Talk was anything like "brainwashing." I responded that Self-Talk is precisely the *opposite*.

The opposite of brainwashing techniques of any kind would certainly entail a method of self-control whereby you would be able to stop anyone who was trying to control you from exercising any control over your mind in any way. Self-Talk not only stops others from controlling our thoughts and ideas, it also stops our own harmful past programs from doing exactly the same thing.

Self-Talk is also not any kind of theology or political ideology, and it is not so-called "neurolinguistic programming," or "NLP." In fact, it is nothing of the kind.

WHAT SELF-TALK IS

Self-Talk is, instead, *the natural programming process of the human brain*—pure and simple. It is a process that is neurological and biological—chemical and electrical. It is a process that puts you in control of your own programs. What you choose to do with that process is entirely up to you.

Throughout the past decade many thousands of people have adopted Self-Talk techniques and have used them to help with weight problems. But it has been during the past three or four years that special attention has been focused on Self-Talk for weight control. Now, along with all the individuals who have used Self-Talk personally, Self-Talk is also being used and recommended by medical doctors for their patients with weight problems, and by professional weight-loss clinics to augment their own weight-loss programs for their clients.

The reason that Self-Talk for weight control has suddenly exploded into the popular limelight is because the general weight-conscious populace has recently come to recognize that the real cause for weight problems must lie more in the *human brain* than in the *diets* we've been trying to use.

AN IDEA WHOSE TIME HAS COME

Self-Talk is the only solution to losing weight we've ever found that is based on the neuron structure of the human brain. And in that, it is clearly different. Though I first discovered Self-Talk in an early form more than fifteen years ago, that difference has now become more pronounced than ever.

Now, when people learn that there is a process called "Self-Talk" they can use to reprogram their own mental computers for themselves, they are anxious to put the ideas into practice. Self-Talk makes very practical sense, and we are ready for a solution that makes sense. It is a *logical* concept, one that is based on neurological fact. Each year, new research is teaching us more about why Self-Talk works, and how each of us can use Self-Talk to make important changes in our own lives.

Many people over the past decade have also used Self-Talk for such focus areas as pre-school and child development, "at risk" children and teenagers, all areas of self-esteem, marriage and family and other relationship problems, work-related behavior and attitudes, financial problems, and a host of other personal growth issues that are directly affected by an individual's programming. And Self-Talk continues to be used today in classrooms, in homes and businesses, in churches and hospitals—everywhere there are people who want to improve themselves and get in control of their lives.

But meanwhile, for those of us who are interested in getting rid of our extra weight, and keeping it off—*permanently*—Self-Talk is rapidly becoming the *weight-control* "tool" that we have been looking for. We now believe that to control weight permanently, the proper use of Self-Talk may be *essential*.

WHY SELF-TALK WORKS FOR CONTROLLING YOUR WEIGHT

Self-Talk has become widely used for weight problems, as well as dealing with many other areas of our lives, because it *works*. But it is *why* Self-Talk works that makes it so attractive.

1. Self-Talk works for weight control because it is completely natural.

We all use "self-talk." We haven't always used the right *kind* of Self-Talk, but we have been busy programming ourselves since our earliest years of childhood.

Now that we understand how this natural programming process works, we have learned how to do it ourselves. In so doing, we are able to put ourselves in charge of our own programming. And every step of the process is as natural and as healthy and normal as when we learned to say our first words or take our first steps.

I have always been concerned about different self-improvement solutions that asked us to do strange things. Focusing on flashing lights or going into exotic trances to effect a change in our behavior has somehow always seemed oddly out of place in the natural scheme of things. Practicing difficult daily "life-changing" rituals seemed as unnatural to me as eating strange combinations of foods that were not part of a normal life's routine.

I have never strongly spoken out against anyone's particular solution to personal growth, no matter how bizarre some of those methods seemed. And yet, I keep coming back to a very basic point of view. Why not solve our problems in the most natural, and obviously healthy way possible? Should we really need trances and rituals to live our lives to the fullest? It doesn't seem right somehow.

I'm not suggesting that certain rituals or even some very odd dietary practices can't help. But the fact is that most of them don't.

Instead of each of us helping our own marvelous minds enrich our lives in a natural and *lasting* way, we often talk ourselves into believing that some new kind of magic will do the job better. The obvious fact that the magic we are seeking is not *natural* to our everyday lives, and therefore will not work or cannot last, is often overshadowed by our enthusiasm for wanting to find something new. All too often the new magic will turn out to be nothing more than another disappointment—rather than the life-changing miracle we had hoped for.

To me, it made a lot more sense to ask the question, "How do we get programmed in the first place?" And then, "Is there some way we could change those programs ourselves?"

Self-Talk is a way of getting a better set of the right kind of programs. It works *exactly* the same way that we got our other programs in the first place. *Naturally.* Just the way we were designed to.

2.   Self-Talk works for weight control because it replaces your old programs with something better.

I have never found a single weight-loss or personal-growth concept that would last a lifetime, if it did not *first* change the programs that had *caused* the problems in the first place.

We know now that we end up "*becoming*" the programs that we carry with us. We live them out. We think what they think. We do what they lead us to do.

Whatever our *programs* think is true is what *we* think is true. We even fight for that "truth." It might not really be true at all, of course. But to us it *is* true because that is what our programs have told us is true.

Obviously, then, such "truths" as, "*I can lose the weight, but I put it right back on again,*" "*I have no will power,*" "*Everything I eat goes right to my waist,*" or, "*Nothing ever works for me,*" are not really true at all. They are what we may think and what we believe only because that's what our tired, old, inaccurate, self-defeating *programs* think and believe.

No one *wants* to have programs like that. We would all like to get rid of them. But in the past we have tried to solve the problem without even knowing that:

a. The old programs *do* exist and they *are* in control; and

b. Old programs do not "go away" by our reading books or going on diets or just by setting goals.

So we find a new way to lose weight, and we manage to override the old programs *for a while*. If whatever technique or method that we're trying seems to work for a while, we *think* the old programs are gone for good. But then, sooner or later, they come back. And so does the weight.

It would make sense, then, that if you could find a way to actually *replace* the old programs, or even some of them, you would have a much better chance of reaching your goal. Self-Talk does that. When people learn to use Self-Talk in the right way, they take control over their programs. And that is why the changes they make—*after* they have changed the programs—are the changes that last.

When you are working at losing weight and keeping it off, the *permanent* change is the change that counts. The right Self-Talk will help you create that change.

3. Self-Talk works for weight control because it is easy to learn, and easy to use.

This may be the most important reason of all for Self-Talk's success. The fact that Self-Talk is physiological, and based on a natural, life-long process in the brain, is very important. But for most of us, if we want to find a way to change our life or our weight—it has to be easy, or we will not stay with it.

As you will discover in the "Self-Talk Techniques" section that follows, *anyone* can learn Self-Talk and *anyone* can use it. That makes sense, because we are *all* using a form of Self-Talk all of the time already. But now that we understand how it works, we have more control over what our new Self-Talk is—and we've learned how to make it better.

As I researched the many motivational and weight-control methods, it became clear that the better concepts were always the simplest and the easiest. There is a reason for that.

OUR OLD PROGRAMS STOP US FROM DOING ANYTHING THAT IS TOO HARD TO DO

Imagine a highway map that is completely filled with hundreds of highways and interstate expressways, forming a complicated tangle of intersecting roadways—so solid and cemented into place that nothing could move them.

That maze of highways represents just a few of the old program paths that are currently in place, deep inside each of us. Now let's say you want to change something (like your weight) so you set a goal to follow a new weight-loss plan or exercise regimen. To do so you have to step out of the norm. You change some habits, do things differently, or change your schedule or daily routine.

What stops a plan such as this is the maze of old program paths that are already cemented into place in the brain. They are strong to begin with, and they are getting stronger all the time. Those tenacious and powerful programs are tough to override. They are impossible to override for any length of time—*especially if what you are trying to do is difficult or complicated in any way.*

IF IT ISN'T SIMPLE, IT WILL NOT WORK

Strong old programs love to defeat self-help ideas that take too much effort or sacrifice. The result is that once again the old programs win—*and your new dream fails.* It wasn't your fault. The new "solution"—the new weight-loss plan or the new goal—was just too difficult. When pitted against the old programs already in place, the new solution never had a chance.

The use of Self-Talk, on the other hand, makes changing programs so easy and so simple that the old programs do not even notice the changes are taking place. That is the goal of the Self-Talk techniques we have included in this book. The techniques that work best are those that work so simply, and are so easy for you to do, that your old programs do not even *realize* that they are in the process of being replaced.

When you use the new Self-Talk, you're not trying to fool your mind—but you're not sounding the alarm and calling the old programs to arms, either!

The right kind of Self-Talk, used the right way, is quiet . . . subtle . . . almost unnoticed—and incredibly strong. Self-Talk is like a team of new programs, ushered in when the enemy least expects them, making their way through the enemy lines, bringing the old programs to defeat before a warning shot has been fired.

YOU WERE NOT BORN TO FAIL—
YOU WERE BORN TO *SUCCEED*

If you know someone who is critical or negative, that person was not born that way. It is not some inbred fault of character.

If you know someone who argues instead of communicating, it is not the way that person was born to be.

If you know someone who struggles with financial problems, it is not because of some predetermined plan for that person's life to be financially insecure.

If you know someone who is living with a weight problem, in most cases, that person was not born to have an unending problem with weight. If you have that problem yourself, you do not have a character flaw or a fault in your personality—there is nothing "*wrong*" with you.

There are some programs you have received that are getting in your way. But underneath those programs, you're fine. You were born to achieve—not fail. You were born to be in control of your life—not for your life to be in control of you.

If you choose to, you *can* get past those programs, get rid of them, and replace them with programs that work *for* you instead of against you.

You *can* win. And Self-Talk can help.

For more than a decade it has been my goal to find, perfect, and simplify every usable Self-Talk technique we could find. During that time, we have tried and tested every possible means of making the process of changing old programs simpler and easier. And during that time we have witnessed the results those changes have created in the lives of the people who have used the techniques.

Self-Talk makes a difference in people's lives—and in controlling their weight—because Self-Talk changes old programs to help them achieve the results they want.

We hope you enjoy your results as much as we have enjoyed ours.

Part II

Self-Talk Techniques For *Natural* Weight Control

Chapter Eleven

How To Practice Self-Talk For Weight-Loss

Now let's get ready to get in control of the weight. We know the real answer begins with getting rid of *old* programs and replacing them with the right *new* programs. We're going to help you do that.

As we begin our first step of helping you change programs for yourself, we can assume that you have at least a few programs you would like to change or get rid of—maybe *quite* a few of them.

The Self-Talk techniques we've included in the following chapters represent the "state of the art" for learning Self-Talk and changing old programs. We have presented several different techniques you can use. You may choose to use some or all of them.

FAR BEYOND "POSITIVE THINKING"

Many people have imagined learning Self-Talk must be just talking to yourself differently. Without learning more about Self-Talk, or taking the time to practice any of the techniques, some people simply try to talk to themselves more "positively." There's nothing wrong with trying to think and act that way, but changing programs is not done by telling yourself good things now and then or by suddenly deciding to "think positively."

It is an inaccurate belief that "Self-Talk" is the same as "Positive Thinking." Self-Talk—that is, *the complete natural process of changing programs in the brain*—goes far beyond such things as positive thinking. Thinking in a more positive way is an important element, to be sure. But that kind of thinking, done naturally, without effort or force, is the *end* result of good programs—not the beginning.

Trying to think positively means having to work at it. And having to work at it means the programs *underneath* your thinking are not yet really positive programs at all—completely mature programs, in place, and *positively* in control.

The old programs are still there. You can override them for a while, but they always come back. And so, instead of having your natural and automatic thinking style be one that is clear, sharp, full of life, hope, and vision, but practical, in tune, and unstoppable, the best you can do is work at thinking more positively every time the idea comes to mind.

It is important to emphasize that the Self-Talk techniques presented in this section are not intended to create a so-called "Pollyanna Positive" approach to life—or to your future weight and health.

Self-Talk goes far deeper than that. The techniques we are presenting here are designed to help you get at the very *heart* of your programmed beliefs about who you *really* are, and about *every choice you make in the life you're living.*

DIFFERENT THAN DAILY "AFFIRMATIONS"

Self-Talk is also at times confused with something called "affirmations." What I'm referring to are the affirmative statements that many people repeat to themselves—usually as part of a daily practice or a spiritual ritual.

Affirmations are often forms of prayers, stated positively in the present tense, and without a doubt, they *do* affect the person's mind in a positive and helpful way. I have used various kinds of these same affirmations myself, and I know many other people who have made affirmations an important, spiritually uplifting part of their lives.

There is nothing wrong with using affirmations. But many people have stopped far short of the mark because they thought they were changing their programs with a few repeated phrases. Affirmations, by themselves, will *not* change the neuron paths of old programs in the brain, any more than saying a few phrases now and then will teach you a foreign language. That would be like learning the words "Adios," and "Buenos dias," and thinking you speak the Spanish language.

Learning Self-Talk is not simply the practice of repeating a phrase or two to strengthen your spirit or improve your day. Self-Talk is learning a *complete new inner "language" of living*, carefully excising and deleting years of old programs that do not belong, and taking full and final control of the programming processes of your own mind. If you choose, continue to use your affirmations *while* you practice the Self-Talk techniques that follow—but don't rely on affirmations to take the place of *learning* the language of Self-Talk.

LEARNING THE "LANGUAGE" OF SELF-TALK

To help you understand the process of learning Self-Talk, I'll compare it to learning a foreign language.

Many years ago, I was a Spanish-English interpreter for the United States Government. My job was translating the Spanish language for the National Security Agency in Cuba during the Cuban Missile Crisis. Earlier, when I was taught to speak Spanish, it was the goal of my teachers that I learn it so completely and so *automatically* that I could go to another country and speak the new language *without having to think about it*.

At that time, it was particularly important that I know that second language as well as I knew my first; a poor translation could have spelled disaster. And in those days, learning a language was much more difficult than it is today, because we did not have the benefit of cassette tape courses (like the Berlitz method) that could simplify the process of programming in the new language.

Now, years later, we have the benefit of technology on our side, and we've learned a lot about the best ways to make learning a language simpler and easier. In the process, we were also to discover that learning Self-Talk is *exactly* like learning a new language—*it even uses the exact same programming pathways in the brain!*

Learning Self-Talk in the right way is learning a new *internal* language, so completely, so *automatically*, that we use the new language of Self-Talk *without having to think about it*. (Learning Self-Talk is much easier than learning to speak a foreign language, because we already know all the nouns and verbs!)

The process of learning Self-Talk is also very much like the way we learned our *first* language. Think, for a moment, how a small child—let's say a young girl—first learns a language. First, it is spoken to her by the people around her. At the same time, people speak the language to each other, and the child hears them talking.

In time, she is encouraged to repeat certain words that the proud parents wait to hear her say. Not long after her first precious words are spoken, that little girl will be speaking in full sentences. Soon after that, she will be conjugating verbs, putting thoughts into the subjunctive mood, and choosing between alternative adjectives. She will do all this by about the age of three or four years old, and all without her consciously being aware of it.

In all of that there was not one day of school, not one classroom, and not a single hour of formal "instruction." There was only the little girl, with her family around her, going about their lives in their natural way. An infinitely complex and lifelong language was learned, *programmed*, without the little girl ever giving it a single thought. Learning the language was, in fact, so simple, that she never needed to give it any thought at all.

If that little girl could learn that language then, so simply and naturally that she never had to think about it, certainly that same little girl, now grown up, could learn another language without too much extra work. Especially if that new "language" is *Self-Talk*.

WHAT'S BEHIND THE TECHNIQUES

In choosing the Self-Talk techniques we are recommending here, we have made our selection based on the following criteria:

A. *Overall Effectiveness*
B. *Simplicity and Ease of Use*
C. *Enjoyment and Satisfaction*
D. *Speed of Results*
E. *Creates Long-Term Changes in Personal Programs*
F. *Direct or Indirect Results on Weight Control*

Each of the techniques we have included scored high or reasonably high on the list. Some of the techniques, as an example, had a high level of immediate satisfaction (feeling of accomplishment and worth). Others took longer but were rated as more effective overall. We have rated each of the Self-Talk techniques for you so you can more easily choose which of them you'd like to use first.

All of the methods we've outlined for you also meet a stringent list of "rules" or requirements. There are five rules by which we measure all techniques for changing old programs.

For anyone who is serious about getting in control of his or her weight (or changing mental programs for any *other* reason as well), these five rules are *essential* :

THE FIVE RULES OF SELF-TALK
FOR CREATING NEW PROGRAMS

1. To create new programs to control your weight, the new programs must be clear.

We have all heard the term, "*mixed messages.*" Messages that are vague, mixed, or unclear do not work in a computer—and they don't work well in the human brain.

If you want your new programs to be stronger than

your old ones, the new programs must be clear, straight-forward, and simple.

2. To create new programs to control your weight, the new programs must use repetition.

This is how we got our strongest programs in the first place, through repetition. A "message" you receive only once, or only occasionally, will almost never become a strong program. Programs are usually created by first getting the message repeatedly from an outside source. Then, as that program begins to take hold, the same program is repeated again and again—unconsciously—by our own *internal* Self-Talk.

And remember, each time the same program is repeated, that program pathway in the brain gets stronger, like putting another layer of pavement on a highway. A program that is received only occasionally does not become as strong as a program that is used—repeated—frequently.

With enough repetition, the new program created by the Self-Talk will begin to operate on its own. The new program (this time, the *right* program) will begin to go to work for you automatically, without you having to *think* about it—or *consciously* work at it.

This rule also tells us why just reading a book or simply setting a new goal will not actually change any of the neuron highways in the brain.

To change programs—permanently—the new programs have to be repeated. Not just now and then, but frequently enough and in just the right way, so that you stop using the *old* program entirely.

3. To create new programs to control your weight, the new programs have to be strong.

If you want the new program to be strong enough to stick, it has to be strong enough for you to hear it. Whispered messages will not help.

Some people have listened to tape cassettes with so-called "subliminal messages" recorded on them. They hoped that by listening to these "silent" messages, they would change their habits or change their lives. It is an easy enough dream to hope for. After all, the promise of subliminal is that the silent messages will do the job for you, and you don't have to do anything for yourself.

I have been asked many times to write about and discuss the subject of subliminal techniques, and I have for the most part avoided it. There are two reasons for this.

The first reason was that I didn't want to enter the battle that was constantly waging over whether subliminal was "real" or not. That question should be answered scientifically, and the answer is clear:

Audio subliminal messages never reach the brain.

Neurological research shows that any message recorded at ten decibels below audible threshold, or lower (the "below whisper level" of subliminal messages), is not strong enough to generate the sound wave level necessary to vibrate the human eardrum. The result is that *no* sound, or message, is transmitted to the ear. And *no electrical signal at all is transmitted to the brain.* If you can't *hear* it, your brain doesn't receive it. That is neurological fact.

Neurologically, subliminal messages *cannot* change the physical program paths in the brain.

But that's not the only reason I will not recommend the use of subliminal techniques. The second and more important reason is that *it doesn't make any sense*—even if subliminal methods *did* work. The real job we're trying to do is learn how to take control of our lives! Can you imagine taking control of your life, getting in charge once and for all, being strong, confident, and in control—*with hidden whispers?* That's the *opposite* of taking control of your life—taking personal responsibility for yourself.

Can you imagine your favorite coach, at half-time, walking out to the team, and then, so quietly that no one could hear it, whisper, *"let's win the game.?"* If you want to get a message across—*get the message across.* No hidden whispers. No wishful thinking. No life-changes that you're not sure are actually reaching your brain.

If you want to replace your old programs with something better—with the *right* programs—*know what they are.* Be aware of them. Put yourself in charge of them. Stand up, take control of your programs, and take control of your life! Anything less is cheating yourself out of the single most important gift you have ever been given.

You were not born to be silently controlled by messages you cannot even perceive—nor was your brain designed to accept them. You were born to be *aware.* You were born to be alert, active, in tune, and in touch with every choice you make and every path you choose.

If you want to choose the paths that will help you most—the program paths in your own brain—you have to be able to *hear* the new messages you are about to receive.

4. To create new programs to control your weight, the new programs must be tied to a goal.

Think of the maze of old program paths in our illustration of the neuron pathways in the brain. Imagine trying to undo or defeat that tangle of tough old highways with only a single new program path or two. The old programs are too strong. There are too many of them for a few scattered new programs to make any real difference.

Then think of creating a *team* of new programs that are all unified by a common goal—your goal—your objective. Imagine a new set of highways, all clear and strong and straight and true, traveling right past the old programs and defeating them. When you want your new programs to be powerful, tie them to a goal.

5. To create new programs to control your weight, you have to stay with it long enough to let the process work. The key is "duration."

Remember, the process that makes all this work is a chemical process in the brain. When you stop using the old programs—long enough—those old program paths stop receiving the "nutrition" they need to survive. So eventually they lose their strength—and therefore, their control.

Since we know that the breakdown of the old programs does not even *start* until you have stopped using the old programs for at least three weeks or *longer*, then it makes sense that if you want your *new* programs to start taking hold, you have to stay with the right new Self-Talk techniques long enough for the old programs to begin to die out. And then, don't stop there. Stay with it!

Fortunately, the techniques you'll be using won't be difficult. So if you are serious about getting in control of these programs, you should not find it difficult to stay with it. You will probably even enjoy yourself. Once the old programs start to change, life can start to become pretty exciting again.

WHAT IF IT LOOKS TOO EASY?

All Self-Talk techniques are *supposed* to be easy. That's one of the reasons why they work. But some of them could look *too* easy. I have heard people say, when they first hear or try the new Self-Talk, "That's too simple," or "If it's that simple, it couldn't work." We know now that the opposite is true, but it is part of our conditioning to question anything that appears to be too easy.

Advertising has conditioned us to accept the "no pain, no gain" mentality. That may or may not be true for body-building, but it is definitely *not* true for weight control. Natural weight control should *not* be painful, and it should not be difficult.

If any of the techniques in the following chapters look too simple—that's a good sign. That just means they have a real chance of working.

TIME TO GET STARTED

First, I recommend you review each of the Self-Talk techniques we have outlined for you. Our experience over many years has taught us that if you follow the steps, your chances of making Self-Talk work for you are very good. The first step, getting started, is up to you. What you do next could be an incredible first step to a lot more than weight control.

Let us begin.

Chapter Twelve
Self-Talk Technique #1
Monitoring Your Own Self-Talk

We said that the best techniques are always those that are the easiest. This first step is easy and takes almost no time. But it is an important step. It will help you know what your Self-Talk is right now.

Self-Talk Technique #1
"Monitoring Your Own Self-Talk"

Most of our programs, even the strong ones, are hidden so deep we may never find them. That's okay; you don't have to know what all of your old programs are in order to change them. But it will help if you know what *some* of your present programs look like. This first step is called "Monitoring," and it means just that.

Begin by deciding that you are going to monitor your present Self-Talk for the next several days. Here's what you do:

☐ *For the next several days, listen consciously to everything you say out loud.*

Listen to *every* word that comes out of your mouth. Don't try to change any of what you say or make it better; just listen to it. If you had someone follow you around with a steno pad or a tape recorder, what do you suppose the transcript of three of your average speaking days would sound like?

☐ *Keep a Self-Talk Monitor Log.*

Keep a self-talk monitor log in a small notebook you carry with you just for this purpose. You don't have to write down everything you say—it would take a full time stenographer to accomplish that. Just jot down anything that you say that sounds like it could be a self-talk statement of the *old* kind. (The *new* kind of Self-Talk is what we'll be learning later.)

☐ *Watch for the self-talk statements you make about yourself.*

Pay special attention to any comments you make about yourself, comments that describe you or your feelings. Here is a selection of comments taken from one woman's list of statements she monitored herself saying in just one day. I should point out that the woman, Candice, is reasonably successful, has a good career position, and considers herself to have a generally "positive" attitude.

First we selected just those statements that specifically had to do with Candice's weight:

"I don't have a thing to wear that fits."

"I can have a little extra (fat) for breakfast this morning because I'm planning on skipping lunch."

"I can gain weight just by looking at food."

"One little bite isn't going to hurt me."

"I might as well, I've blown my diet already."

"My downfall is chocolate."

"I wasn't going to eat lunch but it's really been a tough morning. I'll make it up at dinner."

"I've got a date tonight with my television set."

"Just one more (potato chip) and I'm going to bed. Well, maybe two more."

Imagine if, instead of saying those things out loud, Candice had to actually *type* the same self-statements into a special computer keyboard that was connected to her subconscious mind. Imagine that these statements were actually specific programming directions that she wanted to have happen. Would she say—or in this case, would she *type in*—the same things?

Listen to some of the *other* self-statements Candice recorded in her monitoring log during the same day. None of these following messages has anything directly to do with Candice's weight, but consider the *kind* of programs these comments suggest are *behind* the words she used:

"I just know it's going to be one of those days."

"This house is always a mess."

"I could never do that (become a regional manager)."

"I'm so disorganized, sometimes I can't remember my own name (laughing)."

"I'm afraid it's just not my luck."

"I always get a cold this time of year."

"Edward (to her twelve-year-old son), you never listen to anyone, especially me."

"I'll never get caught up with all this paperwork."

(Also to son Edward) "You'll be the death of me yet."

"Me get elected chairwoman? You've got to be kidding."

"I guess I wasn't born to have it easy."

"I'm really beat. I don't have the energy I used to."

A few self-monitored statements of negative self-talk like those are not supposed to offer an in-depth analysis of Candice's psyche, of course. But from even that casual glance at the self-talk statements she *did* make, we begin to get an idea of the *kinds* of programs that are hard at work in Candice's computer program center. Until Candice thought about it, she wasn't aware of any of them.

Where does a statement like, *"I just know it's going to be one of those days,"* or *"I'm afraid it's just not my luck,"* actually come from? Or how is it that a woman like Candice, who has great potential, can convince herself that she could not become a manager (something she wants badly to do), or that she does not have the capacity to become organized and in control of her life? Certainly, she's not *trying* to give herself programs that are clearly harmful like these.

Candice's self-talk sounds as though the comments were made without her really thinking about them at all. That's true of all of us. The unwitting self-talk that we use daily is simply the "tip of the iceberg." Her daily unconscious self-talk is like ours; it is a glimpse into the tens of thousands of much larger programs that live and operate deep in all of us.

As we have said, you do not have to know what all of your programs are in order to change them. But monitoring what you are saying—and thinking—will very quickly tell you what some of your programs sound like now.

❏ *Monitor the self-talk of others around you.*

While you're listening to your own self-talk, and writing it down, also pay close attention to the self-talk of people around you. There is no better way to recognize the power of a person's self-talk that to listen to other people, and then measure *their* self-talk, good or bad, against the lives they are leading—or how happy and "successful" they are.

While you are observing this, don't feel obligated to mention people's self-talk to them; just be a good observer. You should find it fascinating enough getting to know the programs that drive the people around you while you're getting to know your own.

WHAT DOES YOUR OWN SELF-TALK MONITOR LOG TELL YOU?

If you do not carry a pocket notebook and write your self-talk down (though I strongly urge you to do so—it will help), make a conscious choice to actually *listen* to *everything* you say for the next three days. Make a list even if it only includes a few samples of your everyday self-talk.

Your Self-Talk Monitor Log may have only as many as a dozen entries. That's not many when you consider you may make hundreds of self-talk statements in two or three days. But even a small list will begin to give you the idea.

☐ *Ask your family or your friends to help you with your list.*

Ask the people close to you to help you, if you like. They will often hear you say things that you aren't aware of saying yourself. If you're planning on tackling your new Self-Talk project privately, you can skip this one. Otherwise, consider asking for outside input.

☐ *Read your list over carefully and ask yourself what it tells you.*

After three days of keeping your Monitor Log, read it over several times to yourself. The results of your list should not be difficult for you to analyze for yourself. The following questions will help:

1. What does your list of your own self-talk statements tell you?

2. Is your self-talk usually self-enhancing or self-effacing? That is, does most of your self-talk build you up, put you down, or let you stay even?

3. Is it the kind of Self-Talk that you would like to actively program into your own computer? Would you type those same statements as life-long directives into your own internal computer terminal?

4. What are the strongest programs that showed up on your list?

5. Did you have any programs that came up more than once?

6. Did any of your self-talk directly or indirectly have to do with your attitudes about weight?

7. Did you find any programs you'd like to change?

We're not looking for an in-depth analysis here—nor is one needed. This is a starter exercise; it is designed to very quickly increase your awareness and your sensitivity to both your own self-talk programs and the programs of the people around you. This Self-Talk "acquainting" technique will take only a few minutes' time, and will quickly increase your awareness of what some of your programs are creating in your life right now.

This first technique is not designed to create long-term changes in your programs. It is, however, an important first step in the right direction.

Our rating for this Self-Talk technique:

Self-Talk Technique #1
"Monitoring Your Own Self-Talk"
(Highest score is 10; lowest score is 0)

A. *Overall Effectiveness* — 10.
B. *Simplicity and Ease of Use* — 10.
C. *Enjoyment and Satisfaction* — 8–10.
D. *Speed of Results* — 10.
E. *Creates Long-Term Changes in Personal Programs* — 1.

F. Direct or Indirect Effect on Weight Control — Indirect but important for long-term changes.

The next Self-Talk technique is also simple to do, and this one only takes a few minutes, one time. We're going to help you find out what your Self-Talk would look like—right now—if all of it were the right kind.

Chapter Thirteen

Self-Talk Technique #2
Turning Your Self-Talk Around

This next technique will tell you what your own self-talk *could* sound like—or perhaps *should* sound like. All you need for this one is the Self-Talk Monitor Log that you made for the previous exercise, and some 3X5 index cards.

Self-Talk Technique #2
"Turning Your Self-Talk Around"

☐ *On each index card, write out a self-talk statement from your Self-Talk Monitor Log.*

A maximum of 18 to 24 cards will do. Write out the *negative* self-talk statements from your monitor log, one statement to a card, one side of the card only. It is important to pay attention to the more positive Self-Talk statements you may have logged down in your notebook, but our purpose here is to look only at those statements that could work *against* you—in any way—and change them. So for now, write down only examples of the "negative" self-talk statements you recorded.

What we're going to do next is use a technique we have often used in Self-Talk workshops. It is a fast way to reshape a few self-directed programs.

❐ *Turn each card over, one by one, and on the reverse side, write exactly the opposite of the statement you originally wrote on the front.*

This simple exercise can be enlightening. To help you get started, here are a few examples you can follow. Notice that in each of these examples we are taking the obviously negative or harmful aspects of the self-talk and turning it around—not just to its more positive form, but in each case to a clearer, stronger, more self-controlled and healthier form:

1. Original self-talk statement (from old programs):
"Everything I eat goes right to my waist."

Change this to new Self-Talk that says:
"I eat only those foods that are healthy and good for me."

2. Original self-talk statement:
"I never have the time I need to get everything done."

Change this to new Self-Talk that says:
"I make sure I have the time to complete everything that is important to me."

3. Original self-talk statement:
"It's too early to have to go to work. I'll get up in a little while."

Change this to new Self-Talk that says:
"I'm awake, alive, full of energy and full of life—and today is a great day to prove it."

The problem with changing old negative self-talk to the new, more "positive" and self-determined Self-Talk, is that at first glance the new version seems too . . . *perfect*—as though we were trying to get ourselves to talk or think in a way that *no one* could live up to. When we first read the statements, we almost have a tendency to shake our head, as though we are kidding ourselves.

Many of our old programs, exactly the kind of programs we would like to get rid of, will get us to look at a sentence of the new kind of Self-Talk and almost ridicule its absurdity. "You're kidding yourself," the old programs tell us. "*Nobody* talks that way—especially not *you*."

But that is immediate proof that the new Self-Talk ought to be taken *very* seriously. After all, if our own negative programs of the past immediately try to get us to *disbelieve* the new Self-Talk, what does that tell us? It tells us that given a chance, the old programs would like to stop us—*right now*, before we ever let the new, *positive* kind of programs try to make their way into our lives.

The more unusual, the more *alive* our new Self-Talk sounds, the more seriously we should take it.

Turn your old self-talk around. Change it. Rewrite it, transform it, and watch the pictures it begins to create— even *thinking* about it being *true* in your life:

4. Original self-talk statement (from old programs):
"*I have trouble reaching my goals.*"

Change this to new Self-Talk that says:
"*I reach every goal I set. I write my plan, I take action, and I reach my goals!*"

5. Original self-talk statement:
"*I don't have a thing to wear that looks good on me.*"

Change this to new Self-Talk that says:
"*I look great! I feel good about myself, and people really like the person I am. I look good and I feel great.*"

6. Original self-talk statement:
"*It's no use. Nothing I do will get rid of the ten extra pounds. Nothing works.*"

Change this to new Self-Talk that says:
"*I can do this! I choose to weigh the healthy, naturally thin weight that I want! I can do it and I'm worth it!*"

You'll notice that in the above illustrations only a couple of the examples shown are about weight, or controlling weight. That is because most of the programs that *cause* our weight problems really have nothing to do with weight or food.

As we have already seen when we looked into the "filing cabinets" in our computer storage centers in Chapter Seven, few of the weight problems any of us have really start with the programs in the filing sections marked, *"Diet," "Food," "Eating,"* or *"Weight."* Most of our weight problems can be traced to other programs like self-esteem; programs that have taken away our sense of personal responsibility; other programs that affect our security, our relationships, our self-confidence; or other deep-seated programs that express themselves in unhealthy nutrition and overeating.

Instead, the *non*-weight-related examples above talked about the time to get things done; being alive and full of energy, and going for it; setting and reaching goals; and choosing and creating the self-esteem to look and feel great. None of those self-talk programs mention weight, but any one of them could manifest itself as weight—and often does.

Now that you have the idea, go through the samples from your own list of the negative form of self-talk and turn each phrase around, just as we have done in the examples.

☐ *Keep your Self-Talk index cards and reread them once each day for several days.*

Just the simple step of rereading your Self-Talk cards for a few days, reminding yourself to begin rephrasing your own self-talk more naturally in the same way, will help you experience the value of living with Self-Talk that works *for* you instead of putting up with the kind that works against you.

I should caution you against adopting the notion that reading Self-Talk cards such as these will transform old programs into new, just by the reading of the cards.

Many people have thought that all they had to do to have a whole new life was write out some properly phrased Self-Talk cards, read them conscientiously for a few weeks, and watch their programs of straw spin their way into programs of pure gold.

A man named Steven recently approached me at a weight-loss talk I was giving. He came up to me afterwards and shook my hand, and thanked me for having introduced him to Self-Talk through a book of mine he'd read earlier. "I've really been working hard at it," he said. "I've seen some very positive changes in my life, but I can tell my old programs haven't changed yet. They're still there."

I asked Steven what he had been doing to effect the change. He told me he had lost some weight, but he had not yet succeeded in reaching his long-term goal.

"I have written out every negative self-talk phrase I ever used about weight," Steven said. "Then I rewrote every one of them the right way, rephrased them in the positive, and I've been reading them off and on for months."

I asked Steven what else he had been doing about his old programs besides reading his re-written Self-Talk cards. "That's it," Steven said. That's about all I've been doing. Isn't that enough?"

I assured him it was no wonder he hadn't met his goal if all he had been doing was reading a few Self-Talk cards each morning. I went on to encourage Steven by telling him that if he had been going to that much effort already, he would have no trouble following the rest of the Self-Talk steps that would help him get the job done.

BY ITSELF, READING SELF-TALK IS NOT *EASY* ENOUGH, *REPEATED* OFTEN ENOUGH, OR *STRONG* ENOUGH TO LAST

Steven isn't the only one who has wanted to believe that just "reading and repeating" changes programs. The fact is that this method *could* work if you could do it long enough each day and stay with it for a long enough period of time to thoroughly outclass the old programs with some non-stop speech-making of your own.

But like most of us, Steven didn't have the time or the dedication that kind of a self-help project would have required in order to be effective. Also, I noticed as he described them to me, too many of the new Self-Talk program phrases Steven had written out had to do with his diet and with food.

I should add, though, that Steven did point out the general overall improvements in his life that had taken place since he had started reading his Self-Talk cards. That was to be expected. Some of the lesser old programs *were* starting to give way to the positive pressure of the new Self-Talk programs Steven was keying into his mental computer. The changes weren't dramatic, but they were there, and they were noticeable.

I have often talked with people like Steven, who tell me the same story. After looking closely into many of these personal experiences, I long ago recognized there are clear benefits to writing out your old self-talk, turning it around, rewriting it, and reading your new Self-Talk to yourself out loud each morning for four or five days, or even longer if you wish.

But we're interested in getting *all* of the job done, not just part of it. By itself, just reading and repeating Self-Talk is not easy enough, repeated often enough, or strong enough to last. The people who rely on reading index cards alone, underestimate the power of programs that are cemented in place and determined to stay that way.

Rewrite your Self-Talk, read and reread the cards for long enough to get the message that *that* is what your Self-Talk *should* sound like. Then start using some of the other Self-Talk techniques that will help you get the rest of the job done.

☐ *Begin immediately editing your own self-talk when you're talking.*

Each time you find yourself about to say something the old way, change the statement to reflect the new programs you wish to create. You don't have to be an expert at translating Self-Talk to begin editing what you say, even as you say it. With a little practice you'll find that not only does it get easier, but in a short time you'll also find yourself beginning to edit your own Self-Talk automatically, and very naturally.

When you do this, not only do you get a much healthier program at that moment, but you give *another* strong message to your own subconscious mind as well. You are literally saying to yourself, *"This is the way I choose to be from here on out; this is the kind of programs I expect you to help me create."*

If that sounds like *you*, giving directions to *you*, it is. Strange as it may sound to you at first, that kind of strong, clear, no-nonsense message to your own internal self is one of the most important steps you can take to begin changing the programs that have gotten in your way.

This second step in this technique will have longer-lasting benefits than writing and reading Self-Talk phrases. The reason is twofold:

1. Editing your own self-talk as you speak is easier to do. It literally takes no time.

2. Once you get into the practice of editing your own self-talk, it becomes a habit in itself, and you end up creating programs that reinforce the positive habit—so the more you do it, the more you do it.

ANOTHER IMPORTANT BENEFIT

Editing your own self-talk *while* you're talking is an important step in beginning to change the old programs. But editing has another, more immediate benefit as well. The effect of speaking it, declaring it, hearing it, and taking action on your new self-directions right now, and throughout the day, every day, ends up changing choices that would otherwise have been made unconsciously—by the old programs. When you practice editing your self-talk, you will find yourself making better choices. You will already begin to exercise more control.

☐ *For a period of seven days, completely stop talking about food.*

People who have a problem with weight spend an excessive amount of time *talking* about food. That "talk" itself makes the problem worse.

As a part of your monitoring practice, begin to "edit out" *all* unnecessary conversation or comments about food. Edit every reference to how it tastes, how hungry you are, how the food looks, when you're going to eat, what food you're going to buy, which foods you miss eating, and so on.

That's not "avoidance," that's just good sense. Watch what happens when you stop "typing" food programs into your brain every day, and start to *deemphasize* and *defocus* the subject of food. Talking about food and eating is a habit. But it is also an unconscious pastime that can add hours of "food" programs to your week.

Most of us are good at changing the subject fast when something comes up that we don't want to talk about. Use that same skill now, with food, every time the thought comes up.

Change the subject. Get off it. Talk about something else! Stop making the desire, the preparation, the eating, and the focus of food a part of your programming. When the thought even comes up, *immediately* put it out of your mind. Replace it with something else. *Change the programs.*

Imagine living an entire week with almost never talking about food. Imagine creating that one simple new habit for yourself. When you change what you say, you change the whole day.

❏ *Use turning your self-talk around as a direct motivational tool to help you control your weight and your attitude each day.*

One of the most important reasons for learning this technique is that it ends up being highly motivational— you end up being a better *self*-motivator. And every time you turn your self-talk around, you get better at it.

Another advantage to this technique is that you get instant results. You get positive attention from other people. You *feel* better every time you make a new Self-Talk statement clearly and with conviction. That's because when you create positive enthusiasm by the way you speak to yourself and to others, you also change the chemicals in your brain that make you feel better. And that's not only good for your state of mind—it's also healthy.

Our rating for this Self-Talk technique:

Self-Talk Technique #2
"Turning Your Self-Talk Around"

A. *Overall Effectiveness — 10*
B. *Simplicity and Ease of Use — 7 on writing, 10 on speaking it.*
C. *Enjoyment and Satisfaction — 10.*
D. *Speed of Results — 8–10*
E. *Creates Long-Term Changes in Personal Programs — 5–6.*
F. *Direct or Indirect Effect on Weight Control — Both direct and indirect, and very helpful. Highly motivating and encouraging.*

Chapter Fourteen
Self-Talk Technique #3
The Self-Talk Workout

What if you don't want to wait until you change your programs permanently to make your days go better? What about right now? What can you do if you want to apply Self-Talk to your life—and your weight goals—right now, tomorrow morning, and for the next weeks?

**Self-Talk Technique #3
"The Self-Talk Workout"**

If your choice was between starting a new diet program and starting a Self-Talk program, I know which of the two I would recommend. I would say start with the right Self-Talk "aerobics." Whichever of the other weight-control techniques you may choose to use, a Self-Talk Workout can get you started, add energy to your day, boost your determination to stay with it, and improve your programs *while* you're getting in control.

The Self-Talk Workout takes a little more time than some of the other techniques that follow, but it literally super-charges your day. When you give yourself clear, focused Self-Talk along with a dynamic and forceful delivery, you change vital attitude-improving chemicals in the brain. So what you feel, mentally and emotionally, as being "up" when you use these techniques, is actually giving yourself a very healthy *chemical* boost.

You'll notice the sample Self-Talk we're using for the following exercises includes Self-Talk that deals both with healthy weight and with other issues that could affect your weight habits right now. We're not going for the long-term effect here; the goal is to boost your day and create a healthy determination to do your absolute best *now*.

☐ *Rewrite or photocopy the following Self-Talk scripts on separate sheets of paper.*

Save these scripts to use with each of the Self-Talk Workout techniques later in this chapter. You will use each of them over a period of time. We'll start with a script of specially written Self-Talk that talks to you— *from* you—about your determination to live up to your best. This is a great script to use to start *any* worthwhile program to improve yourself.

SELF-TALK FOR MY PERSONAL DEVELOPMENT

I choose to improve myself in some way every day.

I have chosen to give myself a clear picture of who I am and how I want to be. I have made the clear decision to create the best in myself.

Because I know what I want, I know what to do. I set good goals, I make good plans, and I carry them out.

I choose to always give myself the time it takes to achieve my goals.

Improving myself comes easily to me.

I like who I am, but I also like getting better. For me, it is natural, automatic, and fun.

Improving myself is really important to me. Living up to my potential is an exciting and rewarding part of my life.

I always look for ideas that work. I read, I listen, I practice, and I learn.

I constantly seek and find new ways to put good ideas to work in my life.

I always keep an open mind. I know that the next great idea could be just around the corner.

I find value in every experience, in every situation, in every individual, and in every opportunity.

I choose to set and achieve specific goals. I write them down. I review them often. And I act on them every day.

I alone am responsible for my own personal growth.

I know what I want. I know where I'm going. I know who I choose to be. And I know that it's all up to me.

Those would be great words to live by for a lifetime, but they are especially great for getting your day started right now, or tomorrow morning.

In a previous chapter I pointed out that when we first

read the words of Self-Talk, the picture they paint for us almost looks too good. But if you're going to take the time to *get* the new programs in the first place, why would you ever want to give yourself anything less than the best? Don't worry if these Self-Talk phrases sound like they expect the best from you. They *do*. Every time you ask for the best from yourself—you'll get more of it.

Here's another sample script of Self-Talk that you'll be using in your Self-Talk Workout. This script gets even closer to your weight goals, because it is a picture of you at your healthy best.

SELF-TALK FOR MY PERSONAL HEALTH

I do everything I need to do to be healthy and fit.

I exercise, and I enjoy it. Healthy exercise is a natural part of my day.

I only eat food that is healthy and nutritious for me, and I always eat the right amount.

Even the thought of food or eating serves only to remind me of my own winning healthiness.

I make sure that I weigh the weight that is best and healthiest for me.

I keep myself fit—and it shows!

Being fit and keeping my body in shape is something I really enjoy working at every day.

Every time I hear the word "health" or the word "fitness," I automatically think of positive health, positive fitness, and a healthy picture of myself.

I recognize that not everything about my health is always under my control. But I choose to always do everything I can and need to do—to create the greatest possible healthiness that I am capable of achieving.

I replace worry with action. Instead of being concerned for my health, I take control of it.

I never put off taking care of myself. When something needs to be done to improve or protect my health—I take action and I get it done.

I recognize that exercise is the natural way to reduce stress in my life.

Instead of letting stress affect me in any negative way, I control it—it never controls me.

I choose my friends. I choose to spend my time with people who care about themselves as much as I care about me.

I choose to have no habits which could be harmful to me in any way.

I create only positive, healthy habits in my life.

I program my own mind to always think and act in the healthiest possible way.

I create more health and fitness for myself by setting fitness goals, writing out a plan of action, and working at it every day. I set my fitness goals and I reach them.

I look good, I feel good, and it shows in everything I say and do. I'm taking charge of my health and my fitness, and it shows.

That is all possible, and it is all practical. That, of course, is *you*. And being that person begins with every step you take today. In the action steps that follow, you'll have the chance to begin putting that kind of Self-Talk into practice immediately.

Here is another sample Self-Talk script. This script deals with what many people believe is the ultimate source of almost *all* weight problems—and most of our *other* problems as well. It is a Self-Talk script on *Self-Esteem*, and it is about the action choices you make that will help you build stronger self-esteem.

SELF-TALK FOR BUILDING SELF-ESTEEM

I build my self-esteem. I talk to myself in just the right way.

I choose to build self-esteem every day.

I always do everything it takes to make sure that my self-esteem is strong, positive, and working for me in the best possible way.

I never put myself down—I always build myself up.

I have strong, positive pride in who I am. I let other people know it, and I let myself know it.

I stand tall. I think sharp, I look good, I'm in control of my life, and I like who I am. That's me—that's who I choose to be.

I allow nothing to stand between me and my most positive self-esteem. I was born to believe in myself in the healthiest possible way—and I do.

I look for and find other people who recognize the value of their own self-worth.

By associating with others whose self-esteem is strong, my own self-esteem grows even stronger.

I always find the best in myself, and I always find the best in others. Finding the best has become a habit to me, and a natural way of life.

Every morning when I awake, I make the conscious choice to feel good about myself all day.

I have learned to say the words of Self-Talk which tell me, "I like myself. I'm glad to be me. Today is my day."

When it comes to building self-esteem, I take action. I put myself in charge of who I am and who I choose to be—and I go for it!

I help other people build their self-esteem too, at every opportunity I have. By helping others build themselves, I build my own self-esteem even more.

I have learned to really like myself and to care about who I am.

I am a wonderful, gifted, beautiful human being, and I am always the first to let myself know it.

Instead of dwelling on what went wrong, I always show myself what goes right.

By finding the positive about myself and my life, I always create more of it.

Right now, today and every day, I give myself the gift of the Self-Talk that says, "I love the person I know I truly am, and I love the life that I now choose to live."

I choose to build my self-esteem—right now, today!

   Those are the sample scripts of Self-Talk that we will begin with. They're pre-written for you, and they're designed to cover the basic Self-Talk programs you'll need for your first Self-Talk Workout.
   The next step will take a few minutes of dedicated time. But on those days when you really want to get your motor running and your chemicals moving, the time you spend on this exercise will be well worth it.

   ❏ *Read these Self-Talk scripts to yourself out loud each day for several days.*

   The purpose of the exercises in the Self-Talk Workout is to create motivation *now*. These exercises are not designed to be used every day for weeks or months as a ritual. Few people could stay with that kind of regimen.
   But for the moment, put some energy into your scripts.

Read the words clearly and as forcefully as you can. Focus on the pictures they create in your mind. Let the most positive emotions you've got add *life* and meaning to the words you're reading.

To do this exercise you may want to go somewhere that is private. I prefer the bathroom or where there is a mirror nearby. If, when you first attempt this exercise, you feel a little funny doing it—especially reading something that sounds this positive out loud—that's okay. Most people feel that way at first.

The best time to do this exercise is the first thing each morning. It sets up your day differently and actually affects the chemical side of your attitudes; those chemicals are going to influence what you do throughout that day.

Doing this will not only indirectly affect your long-term programming, but it will help you right now. In an earlier exercise I suggested that just the reading of your own Self-Talk cards would not accomplish a great deal for you other than helping you become very familiar with using Self-Talk. And if you're like most of us, reading Self-Talk cards may not be something that is easy to stay with.

The difference in this Self-Talk Workout exercise is that the scripts are designed to give you a complete "grouping" of specially written Self-Talk phrases that work best when used together. The sequence the phrases are in improves their effectiveness. If you want to get the strongest immediate response to the Self-Talk, read all three of the scripts out loud, one after another.

❐ *Read the Self-Talk scripts out loud while looking at yourself in a mirror.*

This next step can be very powerful. Imagine yourself

standing in a private place, looking directly into a mirror at fairly close quarters, and reading out loud something that sounds very much like a declaration—a "contract of agreement" between you and yourself. There is something that happens when you read the right Self-Talk to yourself out loud while you're looking into your own eyes. The effect you get from this exercise goes beyond motivating; it can, at times, be almost unnerving.

What they say about your eyes being the windows to your soul is true. When you look into your own eyes while reading the messages of Self-Talk, you see someone in those eyes who knows you very well. It is as though the one in the mirror is actually watching *you*, waiting to see if you will live up to the picture of yourself that you are describing.

That person you see in the mirror, behind those eyes, is the person who holds the key to your success. Reading the words out loud to that person will help you reach that success.

☐ *Rewrite the Self-Talk scripts in your own hand. Then read them again.*

Many people have learned that this technique is well worth the extra investment of time that it calls for. It ties the Self-Talk closer to them; it puts their own life and being into the words on the paper by writing it out themselves.

If you do this, follow the printed scripts. After you have written them out, use your copy of them in the same way you would use the printed scripts. Read them to yourself in the morning, read them out loud, or read them out loud looking into a mirror.

CAN THIS EXERCISE MAKE A DIFFERENCE?

This technique has proved to help many people who have tried it. And it is easy to see why.

Most of us could benefit from having more encouragement in our lives. Some of us could use a lot of it. But we don't always have someone around to give us that special talk, or to motivate us, or to coach us on to our victories. What we do instead is just go about our daily lives in a rather average way. We'd like to make each day better, but we don't really know what to do to make things change in any meaningful way.

Approaching the day with the exceptionally motivating and inspiring words of Self-Talk *does* make a difference. If your interest is solely in working on the problem of weight, the Self-Talk Workout will help your determination and your willpower. If you are interested in improving your day in other ways, the Self-Talk will help you set yourself up to make that day *count.*

The Self-Talk Workout may not be something that you have the time to do every day, but the days you *do* begin with Self-Talk—of the *right* kind—will be among your best.

Our rating for this Self-Talk technique:

Self-Talk Technique #3
"The Self-Talk Workout"

A. *Overall Effectiveness* — 10 *For that day.*
B. *Simplicity and Ease of Use* — 2–4.
C. *Enjoyment and Satisfaction* — 5–10 — *Depends on your attitude.*

D. Speed of Results — 10 — Results are usually immediate and last for several hours.

E. Creates Long-Term Changes in Personal Programs — 1-2.

F. Direct or Indirect Effect on Weight Control — Direct effect on weight-related habits immediately. Good day-starter technique.

Chapter Fifteen
Self-Talk Technique #4
Practicing Situational Self-Talk

What if someone were to tell you that you could get in control of your weight in just ten seconds? Would you believe it?

At first, I would have questioned that idea. But think about what is behind the statement. It *is* true that most of the choices we make about what and how much we eat are very *small* choices.

They are the kind of decisions that we don't even have to really *think* about making—and we make dozens or hundreds of these little ten-second choices every day. And we make most of them when we are approaching food, or when we are eating.

TEN SECONDS TO SUCCESS

It is what our *smallest* choices cause us to do that determines if we end up having a weight problem or not. Victory doesn't come in a single moment; it comes in a hundred little moments throughout the day and along the way.

There is no one grand effort, no one great thing that we do one time to achieve our success. Success with weight comes by adding together hundreds of little *"ten-second choices"* that we live through one by one. And in every single case, we end up making the *right* choice, or the *wrong* choice.

Self-Talk Technique #4
"Practicing Situational Self-Talk"

One of the most helpful tools I have ever found to help us get through those hundreds of moments, one by one, is a technique called *Situational Self-Talk*. I'll show you how it works.

SELF-TALK WHEN WE NEED IT MOST

Not long ago, my wife and I were seated in a restaurant for dinner. Nearby there was a table with a group of six people who were preparing to order.

As each of the guests at that table ordered, I could not help but notice the different "food" conversations that took place. It was especially interesting to note that almost none of the back-and-forth repartee was really intended as conversation. Most of the food comments that were being made were merely intended to *look* like conversation.

The typical comments and questions between them were:

"How do you think the steak is here . . . do you suppose it's on the lean side?"

"I wonder if I dare get the brochette; it's usually more than I can handle,.but I'm always tempted to eat it all."

"I guess I should go careful on the entree; I've got my eye on that dessert tray."

"Everything looks way too good! Well, there goes my diet for another week. . ."

. . . and so on, back and forth around the table. Even during dinner itself, there were frequent comments on how much one ought to eat of this or that, how the extra-rich sauce on the veal was too delicious to pass up, and how sinful some dish was.

This was all especially interesting to me because most of the people at the table also said something about being on some kind of a diet, or appeared to be actively trying to watch their weight. And yet, from the dinner choices that were selected and consumed during the next hour, it would have been difficult for anyone outside the group to recognize that anyone at the table was at all interested in being fit—with one notable exception.

One of the people at the table was a man named Michael. Michael and I had met previously at a book signing, and I knew he was actively engaged in practicing Self-Talk—and in losing weight.

It was obvious that Michael looked at the whole process differently from the others at the table. On three or four occasions I heard him quietly say something while he.was ordering or eating. His conversation was clearly directed more at himself than toward the others seated near him. And the simple comments he spoke had an obvious effect on what Michael ordered and how much he ate.

What Michael had been saying, out loud, were such comments as,

"I only eat exactly what's right for me."

"I really enjoy eating less and living more."

"I choose to be healthy...right now."

"Thank you for offering, but I never eat more than I should."

"That sauce may be great, but I've had enough!"

And with a genuine smile, he had said, *"I love being in control of my life."*

Michael wasn't trying to be different or stand out from the group; he was simply being intelligent and healthy. To Michael, even the *thought* of eating something he shouldn't reminded him once again *how great it was to be healthy.* That's because he was practicing *Situational* Self-Talk, and he knew exactly what to do.

Contrast Michael's comments with what the others at the table were saying. Without even thinking about what they were *really* saying, the others made such comments as: *"Here I go stuffing myself again,"* *"Everything's so good it must be bad for me,"* *"I know I really shouldn't but I guess this once won't hurt,"* and a final comment—my favorite of the evening—*"Now that's a dessert I could die for."* (Given enough opportunity, I suspect that comment could come true.)

USE THE RIGHT SELF-TALK TO DEAL WITH THE SITUATION *NOW!*

Meanwhile, my friend was using a technique almost unnoticed by the others, but powerfully effective for Michael himself—a technique that has saved thousands of people from literally thousands of pounds. It is a technique that with practice becomes so natural you can use it without even thinking about it.

While the other people at the table were talking themselves *into* overindulging, Michael was literally talking himself *out* of it, by using "Situational Self-Talk." It took no extra time for Michael to use this great technique. It was easy, it was simple to do, and most important of all, it *worked*.

This is one of those techniques that works *so* well I am often amazed that everyone isn't already doing it! The conclusion I have come to is that it, too, looks so simple that some people don't believe it could work like it does. A deeper reason, no doubt, is that not everyone understands the powerful programming that is going on when you use Situational Self-Talk on yourself.

What looks to others like nothing more than someone saying—almost passively—a few simple phrases, is actually one of the most worthwhile and truly effective self-programming techniques that we have ever discovered. This one simple technique has been responsible for everything from shedding pounds to saving lives. And literally *anyone* can do it.

If everything you say is a program, and if many programs are direct commands from you—to you—right now, then doesn't it make sense to make sure you're giving yourself the right directions? We would never knowingly type the words, *"I know I'll be sorry tomorrow, but I'm going to eat it anyway,"* into our mental computers. But that is exactly the kind of directive we too often type in. The truth is, we could just as easily, with Situational Self-Talk, type in the exact right directive to ourselves.

Imagine changing every one of those ten-second commands that you give yourself every day. But this time, imagine consciously thinking about the words, changing them around, and rephrasing them in the right way.

And for even more help, instead of just editing your *old* Self-Talk so it comes out right, practice creating a whole new set of directions to yourself. Some of them will work so well and so naturally that in time, like Michael, you will find yourself using them without having to work at it.

☐ *Begin practicing using Situational Self-Talk like:*

"I only eat what's right for me."

"I'm taking control of me—right now!"

"When I set a goal, I stick to it."

"I can do this. This is easy for me."

"I do exactly what's right for me."

"I choose to be healthy—right now!"

"I'm really good at being in control of myself!"

"Right now, I choose to leave the food on the plate."

"I don't need it—and I won't eat it!"

You can use Situational Self-Talk for anything, of course. It doesn't have to be about weight. In fact, the *more* you use it in *other* areas, the better it will work for you in weight control as well.

Start practicing this technique at your next opportunity. Practice creating your own self-directions, but make sure what you say is *exactly* what you want your computer control center to hear. Be absolutely demanding of yourself that you follow these new directions that you give yourself. After a while, the directions themselves become a habit. And the more you use them, the more you will automatically *follow* the directions.

Using this Self-Talk technique seldom takes longer than a few seconds. Like a lot of other people who have tried it, you will quickly recognize that losing weight and keeping it off is not the major battle we had thought it to be. It is a lot of *little* moments, the smallest skirmishes of will and self-control. If you want to succeed, you will.

Give yourself ten seconds—*as many times a day as it takes*—to be successful.

Our rating for this Self-Talk technique:

Self-Talk Technique #4
"Practicing Situational Self-Talk"

A. *Overall Effectiveness — 10 with practice.*
B. *Simplicity and Ease of Use — 9–10.*
C. *Enjoyment and Satisfaction — 8–10.*
D. *Speed of Results — 10 — With practice, results are immediate.*
E. *Creates Long-Term Changes in Personal Programs — 5–6.*
F. *Direct or Indirect Effect on Weight Control — Direct effect on weight-related habits immediately.*

Chapter Sixteen
Self-Talk Technique #5 Listening To Self-Talk

This is an important technique if you're interested in long-term change—if you want to do something now that will help you *now*, but also help you fix the problem permanently. This technique is also one of the best we have found to greatly improve motivation and will power.

Self-Talk Technique #5
"Listening To Self-Talk"

People have been using cassette tapes to learn Self-Talk for a long time. After more than a decade of Self-Talk tape listening, it's hard for some of us to remember a time when this tool was not around.

This Self-Talk technique started almost by accident, but it has played a significant role in my life now for over fourteen years. Although these days Self-Talk tapes are used for every conceivable area of self-help, it was my own problem with weight that started it all.

For many years I lived with a difficult and—I believed—endless weight problem. I would lose weight but I would gain it back again. I tried every diet I could find. Finally, in desperation, I even enrolled in a weight clinic, thinking that was my only remaining chance at looking good and feeling good again.

I will never forget starting every weekday morning weighing in at that clinic, getting pills, taking vitamin shots, starting my day in a lineup of overweight people, and feeling miserable. I would take weight off and then put more back on, take it off, and put more on.

At that time, Self-Talk was still in its infancy. I was doing the original pioneering work in Self-Talk several years before writing my first book on the subject, and I was impressed with what I was discovering even then. In those days Self-Talk was being used by only three groups of people—Olympic athletes, commercial airline pilots, and NASA astronauts.

No one at that time had ever suggested that one day people would be using Self-Talk to improve their marriages or earn more income or build self-esteem, or any of the many areas that Self-Talk is being used for today. Certainly, no one suggested that one day people in the United States and all over the world would be using Self-Talk as a major tool for keeping weight off.

But the more I studied the subject of Self-Talk and the growing field of motivational psychology, the more it became clear to me that Self-Talk was destined to do far more than help us send astronauts to the moon or win gold medals at the Olympics. *"What about the rest of us?"* I wondered. "If we took the time to learn how to use it properly, what could Self-Talk do for us?"

I had already spent several years studying the natural programming process of Self-Talk, and I had spent over three years working on how the actual "scripting" of Self-Talk had to be worded.

I knew that if the new Self-Talk programs were clear enough, and strong enough, and repeated just so, tied to a goal, and stayed with for a long enough period of time, the new programs would stick: the Self-Talk would get programmed in and it would stay there. I also knew that if a new program, worded carelessly or in the wrong way, were introduced as Self-Talk, that new—*incorrect*—program would *also* stick.

PUTTING SELF-TALK INTO PRACTICE

It was at that time in my life that I decided I had to do something about my own weight problem, and I wanted something that was final. I was constantly frustrated with living through the trial and error "yo-yo" effect of countless temporary diets and so-called final solutions. It began to occur to me that the final "solution" itself would have to have something to do with the mental programs I had been carrying around with me.

So I got an idea.

Although it turned out not to be so, I thought it was a very bright idea at the time. I decided to write out the right kind of Self-Talk on stacks of 3X5 cards, and tape them in neat rows, around and around my mirror where I shaved each morning, leaving a small space in the mirror big enough for me to see to shave. My dressing mirror was the large two-sink kind, and I covered that mirror with literally *dozens* of Self-Talk cards.

I knew how to write the new Self-Talk phrases exactly right, and I knew that facing me on the mirror each morning would be precisely the programs I would need to achieve my goal.

Most of the Self-Talk I wrote then had little to do with food or diets, or even "weight" itself. I already knew the real cause of the weight problem was buried else-where—in my program files that had to do with old self-esteem, and in other areas. And once posted on my mirror, I knew this new Self-Talk should give me exactly the kind of programs I really needed to change my overweight world.

TRYING TO MAKE IT WORK

And so I began. I set my goal to lose fifty pounds, at about two or three pounds a week, while I followed my other goal: to faithfully read through all of my new Self-Talk cards each morning and each night for the next five or six months.

The first morning I got up, faced my mirror, and while shaving, began my reading of the fabulous new Self-Talk programs out loud, stating and restating each carefully-crafted phrase in just the right way. I pictured each thought in my mind as I spoke the words. I projected the phrases with poetic emphasis and filled each thought with determination and feeling.

And sure enough, something happened; *I got late for work*. But I had set a goal, so the next morning I got up and tried it again. I followed the plan, paced carefully again through each specially written phrase of the Self-Talk, repeated it just right—and got late for work again! I tried to stay with that first Self-Talk goal. But then, as you might guess, the old programs put a stop to it. It was too difficult, too time-consuming, *too out of the ordinary* for it to work for long.

Anything that is too hard to do simply gives our old programs a chance to come back in and stop us. That's one of the reasons that anything we do to change our programs long-term, has to be natural enough that the old programs won't stop us even before we get started.

I could have been trying to work out on a rowing machine or pedal twenty miles on a stationary bicycle each morning. *The old programs would have worked just as hard to stop me.* At any rate, my bright idea did not work.

I was disappointed, of course, but I was determined not to give up. I was *convinced* there had to be a way to program my Self-Talk without putting myself through a morning regimen that was impossible to follow.

I considered having someone else read the Self-Talk to me, like having a personal trainer or coach helping motivate me every morning. But I didn't think my wife, at that time, would look forward to becoming a physical trainer/weight counselor/motivator for twenty minutes every day.

For a time I tried memorizing the Self-Talk, thinking that once I had committed the words and phrases to memory, I could deliver a morning soliloquy of Self-Talk that would surely sink in to my subconscious mind and deliver me from my tribulations forever. But that worked no better than the reading ritual; trying to memorize the Self-Talk was harder still.

THERE HAD TO BE AN EASIER WAY

Because of all the difficulties I had, I finally decided there had to be an easier way. If there wasn't, I believed, I might never find the solution I was looking for. And it was in looking for an easier way that I finally came upon the idea of putting Self-Talk on tape. "I have tried all of the hard ways to control my weight, and none of them have worked," I reasoned. "Maybe what I need, maybe what we *all* need, is an *easy* way out."

My reasoning about the tapes was very straight-forward: We already knew Self-Talk worked. It had to, because it worked the same way the brain was designed to get programmed in the first place. But the process would have to be so simple that literally anyone could do it. I further reasoned that the new Self-Talk would have to be learned without having to work at it, naturally, just like we had gotten our earlier programs in the first place.

Although at the time no one was using cassettes for anything like Self-Talk, it was clear to me that the idea of putting the right Self-Talk on tape seemed to be a perfect solution to the problem.

As it turned out, I was right. I first tried recording the Self-Talk myself, in my own voice, but eventually I took all of the Self-Talk to a professional recording studio and told the engineer I wanted to have it all recorded in a professional voice—not my own. I already suspected then what I learned later to be true. In fact, during the following years, while I continued to work with Self-Talk and teach it to others, we learned an important new rule: *never, ever, listen to Self-Talk—on tape—in your own voice*. There are two important reasons for this:

The first is that you grow up listening to outside voices of authority and the opinions of others before your own.

The second reason is even more important. Every time you listen to Self-Talk in your own voice on a tape, *you are literally opening up the same old program files that you are trying to close up and get rid of!*

When you listen to your own voice played back to you, you automatically tend to be *critical* of how you sound. (What does *that* tell you about your old programs?) On tape, you don't sound like you think you *should*. Instead of hearing the *right* new Self-Talk messages, you instead begin to focus on the imperfections in your own recorded words. Hearing yourself while you are just talking is different than hearing your *recorded* voice. It is that "outside" mechanical sound of your own voice on tape that works against you.

A PROFESSIONAL SOLUTION THAT WORKS

In my own case, I finally got the professionally recorded tapes and set a day to begin. This time I set a different kind of goal. I simply agreed with myself to play the tapes each day, and listen. Anything beyond that would have to be up to the tapes themselves.

So once again I got up the first morning with the goal to start my day with Self-Talk. But this time, instead of trying to follow a difficult regimen, I put the first tape into a small cassette player on the counter top in my bathroom, and pressed the button marked "Play."

I did not get late for work that morning—or any of the mornings that followed. I shaved, got ready, and went about my day. I didn't spend any extra time or make my listening a difficult task. I simply listened.

I played the new Self-Talk tapes each morning. I listened to them at night, just before I went to sleep, and when I could during the day. I let the tapes play mostly in the background, and after awhile, I even forgot to focus on them or notice them at all. They were just there, playing quietly as I got ready for my day or went about my life.

Meanwhile, the Self-Talk they contained began to become a part of my life. At first it became a part of my *thinking*, and then *the things I said*, and then, almost without my noticing it, the new Self-Talk became a part of my *actions*.

What was taking place, I observed, was exactly what happens when we are children, learning things for the first time—like the young girl I mentioned who learns her language first by hearing, without even thinking about it; then by speaking, until, in time, without even trying to learn them, the words she heard become a permanent part of her life.

During the next ten and a half weeks I lost *fifty-eight* pounds—shaving—and listening to Self-Talk on tapes! In listening to Self-Talk, a whole new world opened up for me.

That's a lot of weight to lose that fast, and I would not necessarily recommend that rapid a loss. To make sure I was staying healthy in the process, I went to my doctor frequently, and I made it a point to follow his advice. I even received a whispered telephone call from the doctor's receptionist after I got home from my last visit. She wanted to know what *diet* I was on, so she could use it herself!

I was impressed with my results, of course. Never had I experienced that kind of healthy weight control. But what *really* impressed me was that during the same ten-and-a-half weeks I was listening to the tapes, my then wife was putting on her makeup at the other end of the same mirror each morning. And during the same ten and a half weeks, *she lost twenty-five pounds eavesdropping on my cassettes*.

In my own story, I learned that with the right Self-Talk, used in the right way, I had changed.

It was a simple thing. It didn't take any extra effort to listen to the tapes, and for the first time it took less effort to work at losing the weight. But the most important part of the story is that the weight went away, and it never came back. That was fifteen years ago. I weigh less today than I did then. And I have never been on a diet since.

LISTENING TO SELF-TALK IS SOMETHING YOU SHOULD TRY FOR YOURSELF

Not everyone will choose to listen to Self-Talk on tapes. Some people never get around to it. Others find it hard to believe that any of the more "high-tech" ideas, like audio cassettes, will ever help. I can understand that. I have been a skeptic myself, and I, too, was cautious until I saw the results with my own weight.

Then, too, during the past ten years the whole idea of listening to self-improvement tapes has become a popular pastime, and we have been given a lot of promises. And too many of the tapes sounded so much like each other that we came away with the idea that if we'd heard one of them, we'd heard them all. How could Self-Talk on tapes be any different?

Yet Self-Talk on tape *is* different. What you hear on a Self-Talk tape is nothing like we are used to hearing on typical motivational tape programs. Self-Talk tapes are, instead, word for word phrases of a *new language*—except the "new" language is actually the new programs of Self-Talk. So what you hear are the precise kinds of programs you *should* have been getting in the first place— like starting over again, but this time getting it right.

If you could, right now, type completely new programs into your own subconscious mind, but this time create the programs that would build your self-esteem and put *you* firmly in control, the Self-Talk on the tapes is exactly what your new programs would sound like.

In fact, not only is learning the new Self-Talk just by listening to it a good idea, but it is the *best* of the tools we have found to put Self-Talk into practice—both easily and rapidly.

And therein lies the problem.

GETTING SELF-TALK TO THE PEOPLE WHO WANT TO USE IT

For a long time it did not seem fair to me that the one solution we knew to be the *best* solution would be listening to Self-Talk on tapes. Tape listening was, at that time, not something that was immediately available to everybody.

So for some time this remarkably *effective* technique of changing our programs by listening to Self-Talk, while it made a great deal of sense, left me in a quandary. I knew I had found the answer I was looking for, but how could I get that answer into the hands of other people, just like me, who needed it most? I wanted the solution to be something that was easily available to *everyone*.

I also wanted to avoid recommending any Self-Talk techniques that cost anything—even if it was only a small amount. I knew that would only give some people an excuse to put off doing anything with the idea—no matter *how* good the idea was.

And I felt great concern about people seeing Self-Talk only as a commercial idea. There were already too many ideas making the rounds that seemed to be more concerned with commercial appeal than results. I had nothing against prosperity—I believed in it. But I had always felt that Self-Talk somehow went beyond all that. To my way of thinking, Self-Talk had the potential to help an awful lot of people—if I could just get it *to* them.

I finally concluded that I would simply present the solutions I had found to an audio cassette publisher. That way the people who wanted to listen to Self-Talk tapes could do so. If the publisher agreed to produce the tapes, they would at least be available to everyone who needed them. The publisher said yes, and the first professionally recorded Self-Talk Cassettes were finally released to the public.

Now, years later, and some half-million or more Self-Talk tape listeners later, I am *still* listening to Self-Talk on tape. I don't have to listen to Self-Talk for weight-loss any more. My problem with weight went away a long time ago. Now I listen to Self-Talk that will help me achieve *other* goals—like having more time in a day, and getting my books written on time.

I do still listen to Self-Talk for weight-loss three times a year. I listen to it at Thanksgiving, I listen to it at Christmas, and I listen to it when we go to my Aunt Harriet's home for dinner. I don't think I really have to, of course. It's just kind of nice to think about how good it feels to be thin.

SOME IMPORTANT HINTS

If you choose to listen to Self-Talk on tape, avoid the effort of trying to record your own tapes, and don't make the mistake of having a friend record them so they will be in another voice. Listening to Self-Talk is easy, but getting the new programs exactly right is a serious matter. Home-made versions often work against you instead of for you. Most people don't have the experience to program the right Self-Talk. That would be like trying to record your own Spanish-language learning tapes, when you don't speak Spanish yet.

If you listen at all, listen to professionally recorded cassettes. To do anything less would be to stop yourself from achieving the results you deserve. The professionally produced tapes are now easy enough to obtain, and their cost is minor in comparison to what they do for you.

If you do decide that you'd like to use tapes, there are some hints that will help you immediately. During the past ten years or more, with so many thousands of Self-Talk tape listeners, we have learned a lot about how to use the tapes. Although the tape publisher supplies a very concise listening guide with the cassettes, the following guidelines will help you get started:

1. Always play the tapes *quietly* in the background, even while you are doing something else. Don't focus or concentrate on the tapes. (This is not like subliminal messages which can't actually be heard or picked up by your brain.) The Self-Talk should be played just loud enough to be heard, but quietly, while you are going about your normal activities.

Listening to Self-Talk on tape should never take a single extra minute out of your day. Remember, the easier you make it, the better it works.

2. There are three special "groups" of Self-Talk tapes. These are "*Morning*," "*Daytime*," and "*Night-time*" tapes.

Listen to the *Morning* tapes as close to when you wake up as possible. They can literally change your day for you that day. They help by creating new programs, but they also affect your mental "chemistry" that day, too.

Listen to the *Night-time* tapes just before you go to sleep or even while you're going to sleep. Most people sleep better and wake up more relaxed. That isn't the main purpose of the Self-Talk, but it's a nice side benefit.

The *Daytime* tapes can be listened to anytime during the day, but driving in the car is a great time and place to listen. Also, just before you eat—or even *while* you're eating, put a tape on and let it play in the background. This simple technique often produces *immediate* results. It's a great way to create instant motivation and will power when you need it most.

3. Don't replace other weight-control techniques just because you start using the tapes. The Self-Talk you get from the tapes should help you do *better* with any good weight control strategy or method. If what you're doing now is working for you, add the tapes and your *other* efforts should work better; it should get easier for you.

4. If you exercise, put a Self-Talk tape on while you're exercising. If you're used to listening to music while you exercise, add a Self-Talk tape even *while* the music is playing, and you'll be adding a whole new boost of motivation.

Listen to Self-Talk while you are walking, running, bicycling, rowing, stair-stepping, or working out in any way. The Self-Talk will work just as well if you listen to it while you're just resting, but if you add Self-Talk to your workout, your workout goes faster and feels easier.

5. You may want to listen to Self-Talk tapes just because they help you lose weight and because you start feeling better about yourself—even if you're not concerned about changing old programs.

Remember, however, the primary purpose of listening

to Self-Talk on tapes is to *change your programs*. The goal is to create permanent change. Self-Talk tapes are not magic, and they are not designed to create overnight miracles. Nothing that is "real" and lasting does.

But if you use the tapes as you are instructed to, they can help you make some very important changes in your weight *and* in the rest of your life. If you'd like to take permanent control of your own programs, the easiest way to practice your new Self-Talk is by listening to it.

Our rating for this Self-Talk technique:

Self-Talk Technique #5
"Listening To Self-Talk"

A. Overall Effectiveness — 10.
B. Simplicity and Ease of Use — 10.
C. Enjoyment and Satisfaction—9–10—Very motivational.
D. Speed of Results — Varies. The first attitude changes usually start during the first few days. Eating habits are affected next. Most important is that this technique is the best we've found for long-term changes.
E. Creates Long-Term Changes in Personal Programs—10.
F. Direct or Indirect Effect on Weight Control — Direct effect on weight-related habits. Can have strong effect on your eating, exercise, attitude, will power, goals, etc.

Note: A catalog listing Self-Talk Cassettes that are currently available, including a special "starter set" of *Self-Talk For Weight Loss* cassettes, can be obtained by contacting the tape publisher directly by calling 1-800-982-8196, or writing to: Self-Talk Information Services, P.O. Box 65659, Tucson, AZ, 85728.

Chapter Seventeen

Winning The Seven Greatest Battles Of Weight-Loss

There may be dozens of problems we face when we are trying to control our weight, but most of the rest of them would be easier to deal with if we could conquer our seven toughest problems. In this chapter we will tackle each of them. They are:

1. *Overeating At Mealtime*

2. *Eating Between Meals*

3. *Being True To Yourself*

4. *Procrastination*

5. *Staying With It*

6. *Feeling Deprived*

7. *Hitting A Plateau*

Somewhere on that list you will probably find the one or two most difficult problems *you* face when you are dealing with your own weight. I'll give you my recommendations for dealing with each of them.

The approach here is "interdisciplinary." That is, I believe in using the best techniques, of any kind, *together*—when that is what the problem calls for. Instead of trying to use Self-Talk *in place of* other methods, I suggest that you practice using Self-Talk with any other tool that works.

As an example, in my speaking engagements and seminars I am often asked my opinion about the popular, nationally-known weight control programs. Some of them I believe in, and may recommend—but along *with* the use of the right kinds of Self-Talk techniques.

1. OVEREATING AT MEALTIME

We have all done it. Some of us do it at every meal. Most of us do it far too often. How do we stop it?

The solution to this one calls for a team effort—a team of answers you can rely on.

☐ *Set a goal, write it down, and reread it every day.*

To solve the problem of overeating, you *have* to have a goal. In all the years I have been working with weight control, I don't know anyone who permanently changed his or her eating habits without setting a clear goal and keeping that goal in sight until the problem went away.

It actually works best to set *three* goals: Set one goal that is the eventual weight you want to weigh, one year from today, and another long-term goal for five years from the present. Set a short-term goal for what you will weigh on the last day of this month. (For help with this, refer to Chapter 23, Self-Talk And Setting Goals.)

Write each of these goals down and post them where you see them the first thing each morning.

❏ *Start your day by using Self-Talk that clearly states your goal.*

Let yourself know what you expect of yourself *today*. If you are serious about reaching your goal, let yourself know it. If you are *not* serious about reaching your goal, don't set one and don't kid yourself.

There's nothing wrong with saying—out loud:

"I have a goal. My goal is to weigh 128 pounds by the last day of this month. Everything I do today will help me reach that goal."

That Self-Talk won't change long-term programs, but it will tell you, each day, what you expect of yourself.

❏ *Practice using Situational Self-Talk at every meal.*

Practicing Situational Self-Talk helps you control what you eat with a lot less effort. You may even find yourself *enjoying* pushing the plate away.

Practicing Situational Self-Talk *while* you're eating will help you control what you do next (every bite you take), and it will also improve the way you feel about yourself. When you do something that boosts your self-esteem, you like yourself more and you automatically feel better about yourself. Feeling that way is a good habit to get into. Also, make sure you take note of it when you feel it.

❏ *Listen to Self-Talk while you're eating.*

If you listen to Self-Talk on tapes, play a tape *before* you eat, or even *while* you're sitting at the table. You won't have to keep doing this for long.

Just play the tapes quietly in the background. You can still talk and carry on your normal dinnertime or lunchtime routine. The Self-Talk suggestions the tapes are quietly giving you will be loud enough to make themselves noticed.

Even after listening during mealtime, perhaps two or three times a week, a brighter mood settles in over the dining table, and the messages from the tapes seem to be there helping you even when you're not playing them.

☐ Count grams of fat.

"Counting" may sound radical to some, but it is a perfectly logical and sensible thing to do. If you want to control what you eat, you have to know what you're eating.

Those who tell us to just ignore what's in the food, and instead, just eat less of it, are ignoring the physiology of the human body, and the psychological traps that can be created by the human mind. People who have problems with weight are almost always able to fool themselves about how much they are actually eating.

If you don't already have one, pick up any good food selection book that includes fat gram charts. Learn to quickly look up foods you're not sure of. To start with, write down your totals for each meal and then for the day. Stay with this until your awareness of the healthy levels of the right foods becomes automatic.

In time, once you have your mealtimes completely and unconsciously under control, you won't have to focus on the fat grams and the percentage of fat in your diet in the same way. You'll just automatically eat what's right, and you'll know the right amount.

2. EATING BETWEEN MEALS

Overeating by eating between meals is a symptom of something else. The underlying problem can be anything from boredom to a lack of fulfillment. But for the moment, we're going to deal just with the symptom itself—overeating by snacking, "cheating," eating out of schedule, or giving in to cravings.

Here are some techniques you can start using immediately:

❑ *Set your three goals, write them down, and read them daily.*

This technique should be used with every one of the problems we are discussing. Your first goal is your weight on the last day of this month. Your next goal is your weight (and measurements, if you choose) in 12 months. Your third goal is your five-year goal.

❑ *Make a decision, right now, to stop using all excess salt.*

This one is not as difficult as it first sounds. Unless your doctor directs you otherwise, starting today, stop putting extra salt on anything you eat.

The reason for this recommendation is not just to get you to reduce your salt intake; it is to get you used to not needing the *taste* of extra salt. A lot of the snacks we think we crave are loaded with salt. When you retrain your taste buds to need less salt taste, you will reduce the craving you have for overly salty snacks—the same foods that are usually high in fat.

❑ *Start using Self-Talk to reprogram your taste for*

healthier, more "natural" tasting foods.

The right Self-Talk can help you with this one. The belief is, "we eat what we like." The fact is, *we like what we eat.*" Whatever we train ourselves to like most, that is what we will want most.

People have said to me, "But I *love* chocolate, and there's nothing I can do about it!" Yet there are whole societies of people who have never been trained to eat chocolate—and none of them ever crave it. It is also true that the more we eat of certain foods, the more of them we think we need.

You're actually very natural at liking foods that are good for you. You were born that way, and it's the natural way for you to be.

❐ *Immediately use "Situational Self-Talk" when you're about to say "yes" to a snack.*

Keeping snacks out of sight helps; keeping them out of the house or away from you completely is even better. Your new Self-Talk will help you build stronger self-control, but meanwhile, get rid of the temptation.

Use Self-Talk when you're at the snack machine, when you're at the store, or when you're standing at the refrigerator.

You don't need to overeat. You're better than that. Put it down or don't pick it up. Walk away from it. You've got the strength and you've got the will. And every time you practice it, you'll get better.

❐ *Substitute a healthy snack for an unhealthy snack.*

This is one of those rules that all of us know. But a lot of people put off doing it, or they don't stay with it long enough to make a habit of it.

The key here is finding the healthier foods, developing a genuine liking for them, reprogramming them *into* your life, and making sure they're available.

You'll find that every time you eat something that helps you, you'll feel better about yourself.

3. BEING TRUE TO YOURSELF

We have all kidded ourselves at times, but you don't have to do that anymore. It's time to be very clear with yourself. Being in control requires truth.

The three times people with weight problems fool themselves most are *when they say they're going to take action and don't, when they weigh themselves, and when they eat.*

Most people who count fat grams *underestimate* the actual quantities of fat they are eating. It's one of those psychological tricks we have learned to play on ourselves. But it's a major stumbling block that you can avoid.

☐ *Measure your food and weigh yourself.*

Good scales do not lie. Trust them.

You need to know what you eat—and more precisely, you need to know what is *in* the food you eat. After all of the arguments, fads, and best-sellers, the truth is plain and simple:

Reduce your fat intake. Stop overeating. Get moderate exercise. You will lose weight.

A stack of diet books and exercise plans cannot get

closer to the truth than that.

Start by measuring the food you eat. A fat gram guide will tell you what is in the food you're eating. A small food scale will tell you how much it weighs. Weigh and measure until you've got it right. After a while you'll be able to size up an entire meal in less than two minutes and a few calculations.

While you're getting started, write the numbers down. Check with any good guide that tells you what weight your body frame should carry, and how many fat grams you require to maintain the weight you want. That's basic groundwork for any good weight program.

Next, make sure you have a bathroom scale that works. If it isn't accurate, or if it is not consistent, you will be tempted to tell yourself what you *want* to hear instead of what you ought to hear.

I use a mid-size "doctor's scale." A good scale of this kind costs no more than a few extra dinners, and it is well worth it.

If you have a goal to reach and maintain a certain weight, you should know what you weigh now. Then track your weight daily, if you wish, or weekly. If you use a daily chart, you can expect it to jump up and down erratically at times. Don't worry about that. What you're looking for is a trend. Don't gauge the trend by looking at two or three days. Measure your results by looking at two or three weeks.

Remember, when it comes to telling yourself the truth so you know where you stand, the tendency is to fool ourselves in our favor—that is, to make things look a little better than they really are. That would mean we might "think" we are only eating 35 grams of fat when the actual count, if measured by someone watching us, might have been 42 grams of fat. Keep an eye on this one. If you are taking the time to know what you eat, you might as well get it right.

If you really want to be in control of your weight—and your life—making sure you never kid yourself about what you eat can make a real difference.

4. PROCRASTINATION (GETTING STARTED)

This problem is caused almost entirely by old programs—usually a lot of them. And almost none of them has anything to do with weight.

To get past putting things off, there are two things you can do that will help. The first is to take action *now*. The second is to work on the deeper programs that caused the procrastination in the first place.

To help you get started, we will focus on what you can do right now to *override* the programs that could cause you to put things off.

☐ *Write down the action steps you want to take each day.*

Start each morning by *making the decision* to take action. If you want to get in control of your weight, you first have to make a commitment to begin.

Most of the procrastination we engage in can be turned into action by changing what we do during the first, *vital* ten minutes of our day.

During the first few minutes of tomorrow morning, list a few—no more than two or three—immediate weight-loss goals for that day.

Next, read through your list—and make the *decision* to act on each of the items you've written down. Your chances of taking action—*that day*—are much greater than if you leave your choices to chance.

This technique is one of the oldest time management techniques known, and it works. But now try the same technique again—while you're beginning to practice your new Self-Talk.

The more you get busy with a full-scale Self-Talk program—actively using all of the techniques—the less chance procrastination will have of stopping you. Practicing Self-Talk and *"taking action"* go hand in hand.

A helpful hint: along with practicing the Self-Talk, make setting your new goals (Chapter 23) your *first* priority.

5. STAYING WITH IT

Less than 5% of all people who start a weight control program *stay with it for even one year*. The reason most people fail is because their old programs cause them to fail. When I explored the reasons for this, I turned my attention to the methods themselves. I suspected that the diets and systems *themselves* might be contributing to our problem.

In time I reached the conclusion that should have been obvious right from the start, and it led to what I now believe to be one of the most absolute rules of weight control:

Any weight program that you do not intend to follow for a minimum of five to ten years, will fail.

That means if you start any nutritional plan, exercise program, or other weight control method that you cannot see yourself using and enjoying in about the same way *five or ten years down the road*, you *will* eventually stop doing it.

If you stop doing it, you will revert to what you did before. And in almost all cases, *the weight will come back*.

There are literally dozens of diet books written by competent authors which prove that unique combinations of foods will affect delicate balances of chemicals in our system—which will, in turn, burn more fat and reduce our weight. What they say is correct. It is physiological, it is medical fact, and they can prove it.

But name three people you know who changed their delicate chemical balances and burned fat by eating unique combinations of foods—and who continued to do so *longer than three years*—or two years, or even one.

I'll never forget the time when an acquaintance of mine took off 45 pounds by fasting and drinking nothing but a popular liquid protein diet. It took him only nine or ten weeks to take the weight off. It took him less than a year to put all of it back on again. And he continued to fight his weight problem for years afterward.

What could have made him think doing something that unusual would ever last? He was desperate, I know. But hindsight tells us it could not possibly have worked. It broke the first rule of permanent weight control. He tried to do something that he could not continue to do.

THE DIFFERENCE BETWEEN "WORKING OUT" AND WEIGHT CONTROL

In our quest to find a new solution, we also confuse many methods of "working out" with "weight control." I don't have anything against engaging in safe, rigorous physical fitness routines, but they do nothing to insure *permanent* success with weight.

How many rowing machines, or exercise cycles, or stationary ski machines end up in the garage or store room in a year or two? As a friend of mine put it, "Sooner or later, *all* of them do."

That is not to say there is anything wrong with investing in one of these devices. They can be fun, and they can yield temporary results. But we kid ourselves if we think we'll still be using any of them regularly every day five years or ten years from now. We're not built that way.

The answer, I discovered, lies in the question, "What is the most *natural* thing we can do?" And there are two reliable answers to that question:

A. We *eat*—in the most natural way—based on our hunger and our mood.

B. We *exercise*—in the most natural way—by the way we move most—by *walking*.

If you want to get started and stay with it, only start a program that asks you to do something that is natural.

1. Create *programs* about food that naturally help you eat the right amount, and only those foods that are healthy for you. Practicing Self-Talk will do that.

2. And if you can, *walk*.

If you want to find a weight control program that is so natural that you will be able to adapt to it naturally and easily, and *stay* with it for the rest of your life, *use Self-Talk and walk*.

6. FEELING DEPRIVED

The problem of feeling "deprived" is usually 10% physical and 90% psychological. When we complain of this problem, we don't even say we *are* deprived; we say we *feel* deprived. That kind of feeling doesn't come from a physical hunger; it comes from a hunger of another kind.

The feeling of deprivation that we feel when we are omitting favorite foods from our diet, or cutting down on them, makes us feel less satisfied, less secure and less comfortable with the way our life is going.

As children, we learn to appease our insecurities with food. When we eat something pleasant, we feel more comfortable again for a time, and for the moment we have the feeling that all is well. These feelings are natural; they go all the way back to our earliest ancestors, gathered around the smoking fires in their caves at night.

As the children of modern man, we did much the same thing. As long as we were warm enough and felt full and secure, life was okay. As we grew older, food was often more accessible than personal fulfillment and emotional security. But the food still tasted good, and it filled us up. That habit, though quite natural, was *meant* to be *replaced* with another kind of security and fulfillment—the kind that comes with *maturity* and *personal responsibility*.

The result is that what we lack in complete maturity (something few ever completely find) and what we lack in personal responsibility, we have learned to get elsewhere. And what is the *closest, easiest*, most *immediate*, most *filling*, and most *satisfying* emotional "refill?"

The answer is *food*, of course. But when we feel "deprived," it is not really food we lack. Food is simply the replacement for something else that is missing—and we don't know where to find it.

That is why people eat when they are bored, or lonely, or angry, or hurt, or tired, or frustrated, or without hope. But when you're trying to lose weight, or maintain it, and you can no longer eat what you want, because it isn't good for you or you'll gain weight—deprivation is a natural and easy excuse. To find the answer, we have to look to the cause.

☐ *Right away, begin using or listening to the most uplifting and encouraging Self-Talk available to you.*

This is one of those times when the right Self-Talk makes an immediate difference. In fact, the mood shift we feel when deprivation sets in is actually a chemical shift in the brain. Self-Talk, especially the more uplifting kind, actually changes the chemicals—gets them back to normal, and boosts your mood.

If you have a Self-Talk script of the right kind, read it out loud. If you listen to Self-Talk tapes, play one immediately.

What you are doing is filling in the space that is left by the omission of the food.

Let's say, as an example, that you have an intense desire for chocolate. But, because you choose not to eat it for the sake of your weight goals, you pass it up, and soon after you do, you begin to feel "empty," or unfulfilled. In short, you're feeling deprived.

In this example, either the chocolate itself is taking the place of a childhood-like security that made you feel better, or another similar kind of need was being satisfied for a time.

But now, instead of feeling deprived, or giving in to the craving, you use Self-Talk to help fill in the missing uplift. The Self-Talk replaces the missing fulfillment with an immediate recognition of other pictures of your life that *are* working.

By using the Self-Talk to get your spirits back, and to feel better about yourself immediately, you're not fooling yourself—you're just making sure your mind is doing what it is *supposed* to do for you. Dwelling on deprivation or despair is not a desirable state. Feeling secure and good about yourself is.

Can Self-Talk really replace a certain kind of food—especially something you're used to having? The answer is, yes. It can and it will. In time, when you are completely in control, your system and your nutrition will be balanced, and you'll be able to eat most of what you want. But by then, if you've been listening to the right Self-Talk, what you *want* may not be the same anymore.

Use Self-Talk to help you change your attitude the *minute* you start to feel deprived. And then restate your goal and get a clear picture of it in your mind. The end result of what you're working for will add to your life in every positive way.

7. HITTING A PLATEAU

What should you do when you're doing it right, losing weight, happily on the way to reaching your goal, and then suddenly everything stops working?

First off, be assured that this too is natural. It is your system's way of asking you if you're serious about this. It is saying to you: *"Let's take a break and make sure you really want to do this. Are you certain you want to reach your goal? Do you really want to lose the weight and get feeling better? Are you sure you want to keep working to get those old programs out of the way? Are you still up to it? Okay then, if you are, you'll have to prove it."*

Part of the reason we hit a plateau is metabolic—it is physical, and that means it's chemical. It is supposed to happen.

The other part of the reason is that your old programs are now fighting back. *You are about to get rid of them* and *they don't like that.* After all, they've been in control for years; why should they give in to you now? When that happens—when you feel the old programs fighting back—*that's good news*! That means you have them on the run. Now is *not* the time to stop. Now is the time to have more faith than ever.

☐ *Use Self-Talk that gives you absolute, non-stop determination to succeed.*

What is needed now is not despair. Now more than ever, call on yourself for faith, confidence, patience, and determination. This plateau, too, shall pass. *It has no choice.*

Here's why. If you consume fewer grams of fat than your system needs to operate, you *will* lose weight. Your system has no choice. It may have shifted into a lower gear, trying to burn less fat and run more efficiently because you've been feeding it less, but in time it will have to draw from the fat it has stored up for just such an occasion.

You may have to lower your fat intake, or you may just have to wait it out. Make sure you're getting the right nutrition and the right, healthy exercise. Then look at your calendar, snap your fingers, and before you know it, time will have passed, you will have reached your goal, and your self-esteem will be better than ever.

Let me encourage you. The single most important member of your weight control team is *you.* Right now, you are the coach; you're the leader. It is up to you to create the motivation to see this through.

Remember, if you're hitting a plateau, that *proves* it has already started working! So keep your goals in sight. Don't stop.

You can do this and you know you can. After all, you're really just getting started. You've got a lot of incredible life in front of you. Just look at what you can do — right now, today! You've got everything it takes, so stay with it. Remember, now is your time; today is your day. Make it one of your best!

Chapter Eighteen
Getting Your Self-Talk Right

Getting the most from Self-Talk will depend on getting your *new* Self-Talk *right* in the first place. Years ago, after I had first begun researching the neurological findings that led to Self-Talk, I spent several more years trying to teach people to write their own Self-Talk. Some people took to it and did it well, but most people were too busy to take the time to learn how to write Self-Talk well.

When I first worked with Self-Talk myself, I spent more than three years learning how to word it right—and I'm still making improvements. The reason I have spent years doing this is that the new Self-Talk needs to be worded exactly right. In time I created an entire library of specially written Self-Talk scripts that people could apply to the specific circumstances of their own lives. (These are the special Self-Talk scripts that were professionally recorded and published as the Self-Talk tapes.)

Even without the advantage of listening to Self-Talk on tapes, it will help you if you follow these special scripts as you practice the Self-Talk techniques. I have included the Self-Talk scripts to several of the most popularly used tapes. You may recall from the chapter

on listening to Self-Talk that a listening program con-
sists of special tapes designed for *morning*, a special
selection for listening to during the *daytime*, and a third
group of tapes that are designed to be listened to at
night-time.

The following scripts are from a special "starter set" of
tapes I recorded called *Self-Talk For Weight-Loss*. These
are the exact kinds of scripts that you should use for
practicing any of the Self-Talk techniques.

As you read through each of them, look for the message in the words; look for the actual "program" directions that you are consciously giving to your subconscious mind. Even when you read the scripts to
yourself, you are saying, *"This is me. This is how I
choose to be. These are the programs I choose to add to
my life and give to my future."*

When you start practicing or listening to Self-Talk
that is worded in the right way, you will quickly get past
the fact that it may sound different from your normal
way of talking. You'll notice that the Self-Talk has a
rhythm of its own, with each individual phrase contributing its programs to the pattern, carefully weaving its
message into the fabric of the script.

Here is a script you can begin using with any of the
Self-Talk techniques you choose to practice. These same
words of Self-Talk have been used again and again by
many, many people. Not only have they endured the
test of time, but because of their simplicity and straight-
forward attention to the problem, they have also helped
a lot of people get started right.

GETTING STARTED AND STAYING WITH IT

I have made the decision to take control of myself—and that includes how I look and what I weigh.

I know that every good weight-loss plan starts with a specific, healthy, desired weight, and non-stop, daily determination to reach the goal.

I also know that the real first step is believing in myself, taking control of my life, and seeing myself the way I really want to be.

I know that my weight depends entirely on how I see myself, and what I say when I talk to myself.

I have learned to see myself in a slim, healthy, attractive new way.

More and more each day, I am actually becoming the successful new picture of me that I see in my mind.

I begin each day by concentrating and focusing on becoming my new self.

I set my goals, and I review them each day. I see myself achieving each of them—and I reach them.

I have made the decision to make an important change in my life.

Each day I renew my goal to live right, eat right, and to reach an important personal goal.

My goal is to become the individual I have always dreamed of being.

Getting started being the "me" that I really want to be, is easy for me now.

I know what I want and I know how I want to be.

I am ready and willing to pay the positive price to achieve my goal. And I know that the real price is my willingness to change.

I really enjoy making this new change in my life. Reaching this goal is exciting, energizing, satisfying, and fulfilling.

I am happy with myself for setting the goal, and I am proud of myself for staying with it!

I know that I can reach and maintain any weight goal I set for myself.

I refuse to stop, give up, or give in, even for one day.

I never listen to the negative doubts of others. I have learned to listen instead, only to the positive words they may offer—and to the powerful, positive, winning new words from myself.

Each time I read or hear these words, and visualize their meaning in my mind, I am even more aware of how excited I am to have started on this positive new direction in my life—and how determined I am to stay with it!

Imagine having those messages as *permanent* programs in your brain, so strong and so active on their own, that you follow them without even having to think about them! That is exactly the kind of Self-Talk that replaces the hard work and the struggle—with programs that are *designed* to keep you *naturally* thin.

Here's another script, from the same series. This script is designed to build strong programs of something all of us could use more of—*self-motivation*. Getting *you* to motivate you, usually takes getting rid of the old programs that held you back in the first place. These are precisely the kinds of programs that can help:

SUPER SELF-MOTIVATION

I am my own best motivator!

I keep my energy actively and enthusiastically focused on my goals.

I have a clear picture of what I'm going for. I visualize it. I never let it out of my sight. And I go for it!

I keep myself at my best, and that means I keep myself motivated.

I never believe in just getting by, or doing as little as I can. If I do anything that is important to me, I believe in giving it my best!

I keep myself looking good, feeling good, and taking action! I like myself that way, and that's the way I keep myself.

I am the friend who urges me onward. I am the helper who won't let me stop. I am the believer who pushes me forward. I am the coach who puts me on top.

I give myself daily encouragement. I give myself courage and strong self-belief. I keep myself up, because I never let myself down!

I may be good at motivating others, but I'm even better at motivating myself.

Each morning I look in the mirror, give myself the winning words that put me into action, and create a super day in front of me.

When someone else asks me how I am, I tell the truth about myself: "Today I'm incredible, outstanding, terrific, and I'm going for it!" That's how I am. That's how I choose to be.

I keep myself moving, and I get things done.

I refuse to let problems get me down. I keep my attitude in good shape—and my attitude never lets me down!

I never live my life by following the road signs on someone else's highway. I set my direction, put myself in gear, and follow the inner voice that guides me.

Each time I read or hear these words, and think about their meaning in my mind, I know that I can count on the extra enthusiasm, the super strength, and the winning motivation that I get—from myself!

Those are the kinds of programs we should have had in the first place. Fortunately, those are the kinds of programs you can type into your own computer files now. Practiced and repeated in the right way, those new programs of self-motivation will, in time, become neurologically stronger than the old programs that told you the opposite. And because this new set of programs is about motivation itself, it will help you *stay* motivated while you are working at making the new programs permanent.

If you get good at the above script, those programs will help you stay motivated long enough to get good at the *rest* of the scripts.

Now let's look at another set of programs that could be important to you. This script deals with your programs about the physical side of fitness—healthy exercise. What programs do you have right now about exercise? If you were to sit down and write out your three most common beliefs about exercising, what would they be?

If you would like to install some of the programs that could help your attitudes and your activity when it comes to getting the right amount of good, natural, healthy exercise, here are some programs that can help:

POSITIVE SELF-TALK FOR EXERCISING

I really like being in good shape. I take care of myself, and I keep myself fit.

I enjoy exercising. When I exercise, I can feel myself getting stronger, healthier, and in top condition.

*I set fitness goals for myself, and I follow them.
I keep myself in shape in every way.*

When I set a goal, I reach it. I stay with it, and nothing stops me from doing my best.

I really like the positive effects that exercising creates in my life—and that gives me even more motivation to exercise every day.

I like myself. And I like the fact that I take the time to take care of myself.

I am a great coach! I keep myself up, motivated, enthusiastic, and going for it!

Exercising is good for me. It helps me keep myself in the best shape and in good health.

Exercising keeps me alert, feeling good, and living at my best.

I am proud of how I look, how I feel, how I think, and how I live.

I enjoy the positive feeling of being healthy, and the exhilaration I feel when I'm exercising.

I create a picture of myself the way I choose to be. I set my goal, I see it clearly, I work at it, and I reach it.

169

I do everything I need to do to keep myself healthy, very fit, and feeling good.

I have learned to enjoy exercising itself. But I also visualize in my mind, the benefits that my exercising is creating for me in the rest of my life.

I look good. I feel great. And it shows in everything I do.

I enjoy exercising now more than ever before. I have incredible determination and a non-stop attitude. I exercise—and I like it!

Every time I exercise, I feel even better about myself. I can feel my self-esteem growing even stronger—and I am really proud of myself for the great job I'm doing.

It probably would not surprise you to know that the above Self-Talk script for exercising is one of the most popular Self-Talk tapes that people listen to *while* they exercise. If you walk, work out or exercise in any way, the programs in that script help you shorten the stretch, and "lighten the load."

Another important set of Self-Talk programs are those that kick in every time you sit down at the table. From earliest infancy, we received programs about "food" and "mealtime," and those programs, over the years, reinforce themselves every time we sit down to eat.

Think back once again to the example of the program pathways, the "neuron highways" in the brain. Every time you use the same program again, you lay another coating of asphalt on the old highway—you make it stronger. Each time you sit down at the table, you are about to drive over a well-traveled program highway one

170

more time.

The result is that most of what you do while you are eating, you can do without even thinking about it. In time, the ritual of eating, the things we were told about cleaning our plate or finishing our food, the attractions we develop for one kind of food over another, all of these become programs that grow stronger. In time, it is those programs that control what we do most "naturally" when dinner is served.

Dislodging those old programs can take some time, but when you think about it, it is immediately obvious that unless you *change* the unconscious programs that control your dinnertime, you could struggle with poor habits and badly-programmed food temptations for years, and never break the cycle.

If you read the following Self-Talk script to help you break that cycle, read it again just before you sit down to eat. If you listen to the following Self-Talk on tape, watch what happens when you listen to it *while* you're at the table and starting to eat.

The Self-Talk in the following script also gives you some of the best *Situational* Self-Talk you can ever practice:

SITTING DOWN TO EAT

I am in control of myself in every way—at all times and in all situations.

Whether eating in or eating out, I really enjoy eating less.

I never feel the need to finish the food in front of me. I eat only what is right for me, and never one bite more.

One way to weight loss that's easy and works—is "less food on my plate, and less on my fork."

By ordering less when I eat out, and by serving myself smaller portions at home, I keep myself aware of the importance of staying with my goal.

Every meal, every day, I stay healthy every way.

Less on my plate means less on my waist.

When I sit down to eat, at no time do I allow anyone else to influence, tempt, or discourage me in any negative way.

What I eat, and the goals I reach, are up to me. I give no one the right to hinder or control my success.

I am doing this for myself, for my life, for my future, for my own self-esteem and for my own well-being.

I am never, at any time, tempted to take one bite more than I should.

I am strong. I am capable of reaching my goal, and I am doing it!

Being in situations which put a lot of food in front of me is not a problem to me now. I simply say "no!" to the food, and "yes!" to my success.

I enjoy sitting down to eat. Each time I do, I create a trimmer, happier, more self-confident future in front of me.

Controlling my weight, and my life, is easy for me now. I enjoy smaller portions, smaller bites, and a slower, more relaxed way of eating.

I have set my goal and I am staying with it. I have turned "meal time" into achievement time.

Even the thought of eating something that is not good for me serves to remind me of my own winning healthiness.

Each time I read or hear these words, and visualize their meaning in my mind, I once again see sitting down to eat, in a whole new winning way!

Now I'm in control—and it shows!

There is another set of programs that will help you practice and learn Self-Talk, but it will also help you with something else.

This is a script that helps you take care of yourself, and nurture your own needs, by learning to say "No." Saying no to the wrong food and no to overeating is an obvious choice for life-long weight control—and the following script will help you with that.

But exercising your choice to say "No" is just as important in the rest of your life, as well. As you read through this script, think about the many choices you make each day, and who or what is really in control of those choices. This Self-Talk script is designed to make sure that the one person who is in control of *your* choices is *you:*

LEARNING TO SAY NO

I like being the person that I am.

I like the way I think. I believe in myself. And I respect my decisions and the choices I make.

I take responsibility for myself. I am in control of my own actions in everything that I do.

I respect myself. I respect my values, my thoughts, my ideas, and my actions. I follow the positive, healthy path that I set for myself.

I always say "no" when "no" is the answer I should give.

Not giving in to the demands or the influence of others, makes me even more aware of the freedom and self-control that I have in my life.

My time is important to me. I carefully guard the time I set aside for the things that are important to me.

I say "No" to anything that could work against me in any way.

I have learned to ask myself the question, "What is the best choice for me right now?" The best choice is always the right choice for me.

I say "no" to anything that is not right for me. When I do, I am saying "yes" to success!

I live my life by choice—not chance.

I never, at any time, feel any obligation to do anything I do not honestly choose to do.

People respect me for being myself, and for standing up for what is right for me.

The stronger I am, and the more I live by the decisions that I choose for myself, the happier and healthier I am.

Saying "no" is easy for me. I am confident, self-assured, and in control of myself and my life.

When I say "No!"—I say "Yes!" to my life.

Those are just a few of the program scripts that have helped many people not only lose weight, but get in *control* of their weight, and often the *rest* of their lives as well.

A PATTERN FOR THE REST OF YOUR SELF-TALK TO FOLLOW

These sample scripts are not designed to offer an instant or overnight cure for the problems of weight. But those scripts—those programs—go to the heart of weight control. If you practice them, if you stay with them and make them a natural and automatic part of your life, those new programs—and others like them—can turn years of difficulty and failure into a future of health and success.

These scripts will help you get started with the *right*

Self-Talk. They will help you set a new pattern for the rest of your Self-Talk to follow.

IF YOU WOULD REALLY LIKE TO SUCCEED

If you read and reread your favorite scripts as you begin practicing the techniques, that will help. If you listen to Self-Talk on tapes, like learning a foreign language by listening to Berlitz tapes, the Self-Talk tapes will make it easier and faster for you. If you copy down your favorite Self-Talk from the practice scripts and use these throughout the day, you'll begin to notice a difference.

If you practice using Situational Self-Talk every chance you get, and model your own Self-Talk after the phrases in the scripts, you will begin changing your actions while you take the first steps toward changing your programs.

If you use the techniques and also use the new Self-Talk to keep you motivated while you practice becoming *naturally thin,* your chances will be far greater than if you do nothing at all.

All you have to do is begin. The techniques take little or no time. The "starter" Self-Talk is carefully written out or already recorded for you. All of the steps are designed to be easy for you to follow. And the result is more fun than dieting, and more helpful than exhausting exercise.

In the end, the fact is, if you do it, you will win.

Part III
"Naturally Thin" Techniques To Use With Your Self-Talk

Chapter Nineteen

Beginning To Act Like A "Naturally Thin" Person

Now let's look at what happens when you add Self-Talk techniques to other weight-control techniques or ideas. In this case we will use the "naturally thin" approach developed by Dr. Bob Schwartz, which has been used effectively by many thousands of people. But now add the Self-Talk, and even these already popular methods and ideas take on a more permanent tone.

As an example of this, in this chapter and the following two chapters, you'll hear from Dr. Schwartz himself, as he shares some of his most effective techniques with you.

I encourage you to try the ideas for yourself, just as he suggests. When you do, imagine yourself using these techniques *while* you're changing your programs with Self-Talk. Self-Talk added to other good techniques that are fun to do—in this case, learning to be "naturally thin"— will create even more success for you.

As I pointed out earlier, Dr. Schwartz and I each spent a considerable number of years tackling the problems of weight. We had independently fought weight problems of our own, and had finally overcome them, and we had then gone on to find out what could make the process easier for other people. As Dr. Schwartz said to me one day, years after we had lost our weight and ended our struggles, "Where were these techniques when we needed them?"

He was right. Each of us could have made it much easier on ourselves, and we could have helped a lot of other people a lot earlier if we had known the effectiveness of the Self-Talk techniques when combined with "naturally thin" thinking and other similar methods. Fortunately, we stayed with it and learned the answers, and what we found is helping a lot of people today.

When I first learned of Dr. Schwartz and his work, I was impressed for three reasons. First, his "naturally thin" techniques were based on principles that could help reprogram the user's old programs.

Second, the ideas he had developed were simple and easy to use—so not only did they work, but people could use them in a very natural way.

And third, his approach was filled with an immense love and understanding of real people, and what they go through to feel better about themselves. Dr. Schwartz's caring for you as an individual comes through in everything he says, in each of the techniques he asks you to try. You can tell he's "been there" himself, and you can rely on his guidance.

In this section, Dr. Schwartz presents some of the most popular "naturally thin" techniques for you to try for yourself. When combined with the Self-Talk techniques outlined in the previous chapters, they help you change your habits *and* your attitudes.

Please note that the remainder of this section is presented directly by Dr. Bob Schwartz.

* * * * *

In the previous chapters of this book, Dr. Helmstetter has made it clear that nearly all weight problems are a result of the wrong kinds of programs people carry around with them. After hearing what Dr. Helmstetter had to say, it became clear to me that naturally thin people had different *programs* from those individuals who had problems with weight. And even before I knew that naturally thin people are different because they have different programs, I found out through observation what the naturally thin person's secrets were. These are some of the things I learned:

☐ For almost everyone, being thin is a natural state.

☐ It can be as easy and as natural to lose weight as it is to gain it.

☐ Naturally thin people do four simple things that overweight people don't, and they never diet.

☐ People gain and keep weight for specific reasons, and there are specific ways to get and keep weight off.

☐ You can become and stay thin naturally without effort or struggle and enjoy yourself in the process.

What I discovered wasn't just another list of do's and don't's. It was a way of thinking about food and about eating based on a simple, natural principle. If you begin to practice this principle—this new way of thinking, feeling, and behaving—then you're on the verge of having your naturally thin body back.

It's not weight that's the real problem—it's the mentality behind it. Get rid of the mentality, and the weight comes off by itself, as quickly and naturally as it was put on to begin with.

I know because I lost my weight and kept it off without dieting. So did thousands of people I shared the process with in my weekend workshops, and hundreds of thousands of people who read and used the information from *Diets Don't Work*. So did a special lady named Leah, my wife, who for the last sixteen years has kept off the 40 pounds she lost.

I knew that the "naturally thin" techniques worked, for me and Leah and for thousands of others. But it wasn't until I met Dr. Helmstetter that it became completely clear to me *why* they techniques worked so well. *I was teaching people to reprogram their diet mentality back into a naturally thin mentality!* And that was even before I learned about Self-Talk. If the exercises I taught then worked as well as they did, think how much better they could work when combined with the right Self-Talk techniques!

THE FOUR SECRETS OF
NATURALLY THIN PEOPLE

In Chapter Two, I listed four things that "naturally thin" people do that overweight people don't. In order to change your overweight behavior to naturally thin behavior, it helps to take a closer look at these four "secrets." We'll take the four characteristics one at a time:

1. *Naturally thin people eat only because they're hungry.*

Naturally thin people don't eat because they don't want to do something or because they are feeling anxious, as overweight people often do. Their days don't revolve around food. Sometimes they say, "Oh, I forgot to eat today." The only time overeaters forget to eat is when they are asleep or unconscious, but if naturally thin people aren't hungry, they don't think about food. It isn't an issue in their lives, since they give themselves permission to eat exactly what they want.

It wouldn't occur to them to eat for any of the reasons overweight people do—they eat only because their *bodies* are hungry. They don't waste food by eating more than their bodies need. Food is just food, not love, comfort, sex, or companionship.

2. Naturally thin people eat exactly what they want—exactly what will satisfy them.

Naturally thin people do a funny thing before they sit down to a meal. They usually take the time to ask themselves exactly what would be satisfying to them. They look to see what they want before they start eating.

They don't ask themselves what they shouldn't eat; they ask themselves what they *want* to eat. They seem to have some sort of inner barometer that tells them not only what would taste good at that particular moment, but also what would satisfy their bodies' wants and needs.

They know that if they want a steak, a head of lettuce isn't going to satisfy them. If they really want a baked potato, cottage cheese isn't going to make them happy. If you want chocolate ice cream, even a thousand carrot sticks aren't going to satisfy your craving!

Normally, naturally thin people are finicky eaters—

they don't eat what they don't want. They don't eat just to be eating; they eat because a particular food rings a loud bell for them and because they are hungry.

If they're out to lunch and nothing on the menu sounds tantalizing, either they'll leave and go elsewhere, or they'll order a token serving just to take the edge off their hunger. They do strange things, like not finishing everything on their plates. If a plate containing meat, vegetables, and potatoes is set in front of them, they'll only eat what they like. They may eat just the meat and the spinach, for example, and leave behind a mound of mashed potatoes. Or they may not touch the meat and eat a dessert instead. Sometimes, if they have the option, *they may not eat at all*. They'll do something else instead. *They know there will always be another meal.*

As strange as this principle may sound to someone who has spent years on strict diet plans, I have found it to be one of the quickest shortcuts to better nutrition. What happens is very interesting.

As you begin to eat *exactly* what you want, your body begins to become clear about which foods make you feel naturally thin and energetic and which make you feel bloated and tired. It doesn't take long before you will begin to want *exactly* those foods which are in alignment with your new naturally thin and healthy eating goals. Your new Self-Talk about "eating healthy" begins to support the choices your body is making about which foods are best for you.

3. *Naturally thin people eat consciously and enjoy every bite.*

They are conscious of what they are eating and the effect the food is having on their bodies. *Since they pay attention and enjoy every bite of what they're eating,*

183

they're satisfied with less and enjoy their food more!

Overeaters never get tired of eating because they eat while thinking about everything except the food on their plates, and they seldom even taste their food until the end of a meal.

Because naturally thin people are aware and conscious when they're eating, they know when their body reaches the "not hungry" level. Most overweight people have no idea how hungry they are before they eat, while they're eating, or after they eat. Naturally thin people stay "tuned in" to their bodies, and they know when their bodies aren't hungry anymore.

4. Naturally thin people stop eating when their bodies aren't hungry anymore.

Did you ever have someone try to press more food on you? Naturally thin people have three words that stop people from trying to get them to eat more than they want. They say, *"I'm not hungry,"* and if pressed, they just apologetically keep repeating those three words.

Haven't you seen naturally thin people stop eating right in the middle of an expensive meal, push their plate away, and feel no guilt whatsoever? Have you ever seen them wrap up and save as little as two bites of food, or take all but two sips of a soft drink and put it back in the refrigerator? Have you ever asked them why they don't finish what they are eating or drinking, and hear them say, *"I'm not hungry. I'll finish it later.?"* Doggie bags were invented for naturally thin people. Overweight people eat everything that lands on the table.

Naturally thin people don't care whether or not they're in the Clean Plate Club. They will occasionally overeat, but they don't give occasional overeating a second thought. They treat food as if it were their servant, not their master. They don't pay an *excessive* amount of attention to it, even when they are consciously enjoying what they eat. Sometimes they will ignore the food, leave it sitting on their plate, and even throw it away!

THE BIG DIFFERENCE BETWEEN NATURALLY THIN PEOPLE AND OVERWEIGHT PEOPLE

Suppose you had a naturally thin friend who was heartbroken because she'd just broken up with her boyfriend. As she sat there crying, you reached out in compassion and offered her a donut. What do you suppose she would do?

She would probably look at you and then look at the donut, trying to figure out what you were doing. Perhaps she would ask you if there were some kind of drug in the donut. But no, you assure her it's just a regular donut. At this point she would probably ask in desperation, *"But what am I supposed to do with it?"*

You see, to her food is something you put into your body when you're hungry, the fuel you use to keep your body going. She doesn't understand about food and problem solving. She doesn't confuse physical and emotional hungers.

The big difference between naturally thin people and overweight people is this:

Naturally thin people eat for only one reason: because they're hungry. Overweight people eat for many reasons, most of which have absolutely nothing to do with food or nutrition.

Who are these "naturally thin" people who are so igno-
rant they don't know the number of calories or fat grams
in a chocolate chip cookie, who don't even know what
they do to stay thin? Why are naturally thin people like
that, why are they different from overweight people, and
how did they get that way?

The truth is that they didn't do anything special, and
they don't know anything the rest of us don't. That's
just the point: *being thin is a natural state*. We are the
ones who have done something, who have added something to nature. We're the ones who have created the
myths and the patterns and the rules that make and
keep us overweight. Take those myths and patterns and
rules away, and what you have is a natural state—
naturally thin. The naturally thin people are like animals in the wild, following their bodies' instincts from
moment to moment.

Have you ever asked a naturally thin person why they
eat? Try it a couple of times today. When I've tried it,
the thin person usually eyed me suspiciously and said,
"Is this some kind of trick question?" When I assured
them that I really wanted to know, they looked at me as
if I were crazy and said, *"I eat because I'm hungry, of
course."*

You rarely get that answer from people with weight
problems, and now you can begin to see why. Overweight people find they are so busy eating that they very
seldom get to the point of hunger. By not knowing what
it's like to be hungry, they can't eat only when their
bodies tell them it's time. Overeaters eat because the
food smells good or tastes good, because it might spoil if
they don't eat it, or simply because it's there. They start
to feel like eating machines that someone forgot to turn
off.

Overeaters use food to satisfy all kinds of hunger—

emotional hunger, intellectual hunger, sexual hunger. They feel a feeling and habitually assume it's for food. The problem is that those hungers never really get satisfied by food.

THE BIG THIRTEEN

In *Diets Don't Work* I laid out thirty typical reasons for overeating that the people in my weekend workshops usually came up with. Over the last ten years I have found that the main reasons most people overeat fall into the following thirteen categories. As you read this list for the first time, put a check mark by any of the reasons that trigger *you* to eat or overeat:

1. *Feeling stress or tension.*
2. *Not getting what you want.*
3. *Resisting doing something you don't want to do.*
4. *Hiding your thoughts or feelings from someone.*
5. *Boredom.*
6. *For pleasure.*
7. *Going unconscious (eating automatically).*
8. *Scarcity ("If I don't eat it now, I won't get it later.").*
9. *Unfulfilled sexual or relationship expectations.*
10. *To get approval (making someone happy by eating).*
11. *To avoid feeling any feeling you don't want to feel.*
12. *Feeling incomplete or empty.*
13. *"Grazing"—craving something and eating everything.*

How many of these reasons do you use (or should I say, "Use you?") to overeat?

Naturally Thin Technique #1
"Beginning To Act Like A Naturally Thin Person"

Part 1. For the next three days, carry a notebook with you and write out which specific situations or times you are usually affected by any of these or other reasons for eating or overeating. Each time you "trigger," immediately replace the desire to overeat with the "naturally thin" Self-Talk that says, *"I never feed my emotions with food. I eat only when my body is hungry."*

Each time you do this, you will become more aware of your body's needs, and less likely to eat for reasons other than physical hunger.

Our goal in writing this book, and combining the techniques of Self-Talk with the Naturally Thin techniques, is to *end weight as a problem in your life forever*, so that you can go on to do all those things you were going to do *after* you lost your weight.

Part 2 of this technique will help you begin to discover what your life will be like as a naturally thin person.

Part 2. If you woke up tomorrow morning with a new naturally thin body and were exactly the weight you wanted to be, what three things would you do?

Write out your answers in the spaces provided below (or on a separate sheet of paper). Don't limit your answers to those things you can do *now*, at your current weight. Remember, the key is to begin to picture yourself being naturally thin, and doing the things naturally thin people do. Go ahead and write it down—even if it seems silly or impossible for now.

WHAT I WOULD DO NOW IF I WERE
NATURALLY THIN

1. _____
_____
_____

2. _____
_____
_____

3. _____
_____
_____

As you think of more things to do after you become naturally thin, add to this list. As you continue reading through the book, refer back to this list and begin to act like a naturally thin person by doing the things on your list, one at a time—easiest things first. The key to this technique is for you to stop waiting until you've lost the weight to do the things you've always wanted to do. It is designed to get you to start acting like a naturally thin person now—*while* you are using the Self-Talk techniques to permanently reprogram your weight.

Chapter Twenty
Listening To Your Emotions

Most of the eating habits we've talked about have an emotional dimension. In some cases, the specific purpose of overeating is trying to get rid of feelings, to make them go away by stuffing them down with food.

Stuffing feelings down with food is a game that's difficult to win. You're always going to have feelings, both positive and negative, and if you head for the refrigerator every time you start to have what you consider to be an uncomfortable emotion, you're going to get very heavy in a hurry. If, on the other hand, you can unhook food from your emotions, you accomplish two important things:

☐ Your weight is no longer dependent on how you feel.

☐ You can bring your emotions to the surface, experience them, and do something about them.

In order to have a breakthrough with your weight and eating, you are going to have to begin a new way of thinking, a new way of looking at old problems. As Dr. Helmstetter points out, that change of mental attitude won't happen overnight, but if you combine the Self-Talk Techniques and the Naturally Thin Exercises and stay with them, it *will* happen. Your brain has no choice.

**Naturally Thin Exercise #2
"Listening To Your Emotions"**

The main thing with this technique is to be patient with yourself, give yourself plenty of time, and leave room for error. Learning to .deal with your emotions takes practice, and if you're used to covering up your feelings with food, it may be a bit uncomfortable at first. That's okay—just keep going. And remember to keep your sense of humor; I've never met anyone who became naturally thin by being grim and serious.

WHAT YOUR EMOTIONS ARE TRYING TO TELL YOU

When you feel emotions like anger, hurt, or sadness, and then cover that feeling with food, you never get to the root of the problem. Much of the pain and resentment you feel when you are overweight comes from the inner knowledge that *you deserve better*.

One of the most devastating problems with the mental condition that I named the Diet Mentality is that it encourages you to dislike yourself and your body and to treat yourself accordingly—and you wind up denying yourself the very things that could make you feel better about yourself. It becomes a vicious cycle: you feel bad about yourself, so you fail to do those things that would make you feel loved and appreciated and worthwhile— and then you feel even worse about yourself.

For too long, we've all been indoctrinated—*programmed*—with the idea that we have to use harsh discipline on ourselves to get results. In fact, in the long run, just the opposite is true. The *Naturally Thin* approach to the whole issue of weight-loss is to be kind, positive, and gentle with yourself.

Being overweight is not a crime. The person inside your body, the real you, is a capable and worthy individual, even if you presently don't think so. I invite you to put self-recrimination aside while you try this exercise, and start now to see what it would be like to be loving toward yourself.

There are probably hundreds of ways that you daily deprive yourself or treat yourself like a second-class person. With this exercise, you get to play the part of your best friend, someone who knows everything about you. You're going to list the things that, if someone did them for you, would make you feel cared about.

This is an extremely important exercise. The purpose of it right now is for you to get down in black and white all of the many ways in which you are not now treating yourself like a naturally thin person. Once you see what they are, you can begin to change them, and begin once and for all treating yourself like you truly deserve to be treated.

THINGS YOU WOULD LIKE TO DO FOR YOURSELF THAT WOULD MAKE YOU FEEL CARED ABOUT

In this exercise, you will make three separate lists of things that you'd like to do for yourself, or have done for you, that would make you feel loved, appreciated, and cared about. Fill in each list as follows:

1. Three personal things I would like to do for myself that would make me feel cared about are:

a. _____

_____

b. _____

_____

c. _____

_____

2. Three things I would like to do in my relationships that would make me feel cared about are:

a. _____

_____

b. _____

_____

c. _____

_____

3. Three things I would like to do or have done for my body that would make me feel cared about are:

a. _____

_____

b. _____

_____

c.
_____

_____

Now, take a moment, and go back and read those three categories. This time, even if you aren't stopping right now to write out your lists, think of some of the things you would add to your lists.

Don't think too much when you answer the questions. If you get stuck, just keep writing. Make something up. You will discover when you go back and read over what you have written that some of your "made-up" answers may begin to make a lot of sense. And writing the answers down creates results for you that just thinking about the answers does not.

A LITTLE HELP FROM YOUR FRIENDS

If you are reading this book with someone else who is close to you, such as a spouse or close friend or family member, each of you should write your answers separately. Feel free to keep some or all of your answers private if you feel more comfortable that way.

Doing the exercises together with someone close to you is a great way to learn things about each other—and to let the other person know exactly what they can do to help you start feeling great about yourself, right now! And best of all, you will learn how to support each other in being naturally thin.

Chapter Twenty-One
A Taste Of The Thin Life

The best way for you to learn how naturally thin people operate is to experience a day of approaching food the way they do. In my weekend workshop, I actually serve participants a meal, during which we go through certain exercises to emphasize the Naturally Thin Mentality. I would like you to choose a day of relative freedom, say a Saturday or a Sunday, and create the experience of eating meals the way a naturally thin person would and spend the day in the Naturally Thin Mentality.

Naturally Thin Exercise #3
"A Taste Of the Thin Life"

In order to actually experience the Naturally Thin Mentality, you will need to know several things:

1. Rating Your Hunger.

Since most people who eat too much don't have a very clear idea of what it feels like to be really hungry, I've devised a hunger scale, with 1 at the bottom and 10 at the top.

"One" is when you're so hungry you feel faint. "Ten" is

when you're so stuffed you can hardly move. In the middle, at 5 on the scale—which we will call *not hungry*—is the point at which your body has had enough to eat.

Everything up to 4.99 is "hungry"; everything from 5.01 on up is "overeating," or "too much," what overweight people call "full."

2. *Disconnecting The Eating Machine.*

In order to follow the third principle of naturally thin eating—that is, enjoying the eating of every bite consciously—you have to know how to get yourself off automatic. I call the process "disconnecting the eating machine." The object is to keep your attention on the food that's already in your mouth, so you actually taste and enjoy it.

To achieve this, I have the people in my workshops put their forks down *before* they start to chew. Then I have them completely chew the bites that are in their mouths, squeezing out all the flavor and goodness possible before swallowing it. Only then do they pick up their forks again.

3. *Sizing Up Your Stomach.*

Before we begin the meal at the workshop, I have everyone make a fist with their right hand. *This is the approximate size of your stomach.*

If you're completely empty, the approximate volume of food you need to eat to satisfy your body's hunger might only fill a container about the size of your fist. How many bites of food do you suppose that would be?

4. Rating Food.

Another thing that is useful to know before spending the day as a naturally thin eater is how to rate food. Naturally thin people generally only eat foods they really love. So I've developed a food-rating scale, again from 1 to 10, with the numbers on the bottom of the scale representing your least-favorite foods and those at the top of the scale representing your favorite foods of all time.

Foods at the level of 1 or 2 probably have no business being in your mouth. Naturally thin people generally only eat foods that are 7s, 8s, 9s or 10s for them. This is entirely a matter of taste; everybody has different preferences.

Take a few minutes and think of some foods which would fit in each of these categories for you:

10 Wonderful; fantastic
 9
 8 Pretty good
 7
 6 OK, but not quality
 5
 4 Not good
 3
 2 UGH!
 1

5. Getting In The Mood.

Since you don't have the advantage of being in my workshop room where every aspect of your meal is controlled, you will need to know how to approach eating on your naturally thin day.

First, treat yourself like a naturally thin person for that whole day. When you sit down to eat your meals, pretend you're an honored guest and someone has gone to a great deal of trouble to prepare delicious food for you to eat. In the workshop, we dim the lights in the room and play soft, relaxing music.

You may want to eat alone, so you can concentrate on the process of eating like a naturally thin person without any distractions. If you do eat with someone, make sure that person is participating with you, supporting you in doing the exercise.

6. Doing What Naturally Thin People Do When They're Not Eating.

Make a list of at least 20 things you would really like to do or complete during your first naturally thin day. If you had one whole day to do anything that you wanted, what would you do? Maybe something is bothering you because it is not finished, such as cleaning out and organizing your refrigerator, or calling people with whom you have not talked in a long time.

No matter what you choose to do on your naturally thin day, just make sure that it is going to be fun or it is going to make you feel good. Don't make the projects too complicated. Break them down into easy-to-do steps so that you can have the feeling of winning at each step.

The most important thing to remember is to *make sure you feel like you win with each item you complete, and either make what you are doing fun or have the accomplishment make you feel good that you completed it.*

Don't worry if you don't come close to completing all 20 of your items. That is not the object of this exercise. The point is to pretend to do the things a naturally thin person might do, rather than think about food or weight and to *have fun.*

7. What To Eat?

I want you to make up your own list of foods to eat for your naturally thin day. The only guidelines I want you to follow on your naturally thin day are to avoid alcohol, and don't eat or drink anything except water between meals.

In order to make the exercise a success, choose and make a list of a large variety of foods. Include items you would rank as 7s, 8s, 9s or 10s, as well as "healthy" items for contrast that might be 3s or 4s. Also include a variety of fresh foods, such as raw fruit and vegetables.

Pre-plan exactly what you think you would like to eat and drink during each meal. Remember, you will be sampling a lot of different foods to see what they taste like when eaten by a naturally thin person.

THIN FOR A DAY

Your day has arrived! This is the day you have chosen to be your first-ever Naturally Thin Day—the blueprint for all the wonderful, naturally thin days to follow in your life. You have your list of 20 things you'd like to get done today; you've carefully planned your menus and set aside the time and environment to make today a success. Now, take a deep breath, smile at yourself, and *begin.*

Read through the following procedure, and follow it step by step. (It's a good idea to reread the list before each meal, and refer to it throughout your Naturally

Thin Day.)

1. Wait until you are hungry before you eat each meal. You may not get hungry three times a day, so you may eat less than three meals. It does not make any difference if you eat breakfast food at lunch, or dinner food for breakfast. Eat exactly what you want.

2. Before each meal, check your level of hunger, and write down the number you think it is.

3. Before each meal, set the table and prepare your plate as if you were serving a very special person. (You are!)

4. Sit down and get ready to eat. Before you start, pick up your plate and look at each item as if you had never seen it before. Pretend the food on your plate came from another planet, even though it might look like something you've eaten before.
Next, smell each item. Can you determine from the smell what it might taste like? If you couldn't see the food, what color does it smell like it would be?

5. Start by picking up the most delicious item on your plate with your fingers or your fork; raise it slowly to your nose, and smell the aroma. Next, closely examine what it looks like. Now put the food into your mouth, but before you begin to chew, disconnect the eating machine. Put your fork or the food down on the plate.

6. Before starting to chew, gently savor this morsel of food for a moment. Move it around in your mouth. See if you notice different flavors when moving it to different parts of your mouth.

7. Now bite down on the food. Continue to chew the bite very slowly, and concentrate on enjoying every time your teeth cut through the food.

8. After you've chewed on this bite as much as possible and have swallowed it, notice the taste it leaves in your mouth. Savor the pleasure you can get out of the aftertaste.

9. Now go around the plate, eating one bite of each food in the same manner as you did the first. Select each bite in the order that you would rate them from most favorite to least favorite. Notice if you change your mind about their rating after you've eaten each item like a naturally thin person.

10. After you've tasted every item on the plate once, put your fork down, pause a moment, and look at the food again. Which of the foods were 10s for you, and what numbers would you give the other items?

11. Check your level of hunger before you continue. How much has your hunger level changed since you started?

12. Before you continue, do something your mother told you never to do: *play with your food.*
Rearrange it into a picture of something or make a design out of it.
Mash or mix it up.
Pick up a piece of food and while holding it a foot or two over your plate, "bomb" some target on your plate.
As you play with your food, listen to the voices in your head. If they try to get you to stop, thank them for their advice and *keep going* until you get tired of playing with

your food. Is the food starting to lose some of its emotional charge and become just food?

13. Continue the meal to satisfy your remaining hunger. Eat slowly, and put your fork down before beginning to chew. Eat only the remaining foods on the plate that are 7s, 8s, 9s, or 10s for you.

14. As you complete the meal, keep checking your level of hunger. If you're not sure whether your body is at level 5 (not hungry), give yourself permission to eat three more bites, then stop for a moment, check your hunger level again, and continue if still hungry.

15. This next step may be very hard for you. Just keep breathing and stay in touch with what you are feeling and thinking.
When you reach "not hungry," pick up your plate, carry it to the garbage can, and very slowly *discard the remaining food*. Notice how you feel about throwing food away instead of stuffing it into your body.

16. After each meal, spend about five minutes just thinking quietly about your experience. Write down your impressions of what eating like a naturally thin person was like for you after each meal.

17. After your first meal, instead of throwing any leftover food away (except for the remainder on your plate, as discussed in step 15), wrap some of the parts worth saving for tomorrow.

18. After each meal is complete, refer to the list of things that you wanted to accomplish today. Pick the one which is the most important or the one that you

would most like to do. Begin to work on that project, and be aware of how good you feel as you complete each step.

19. Do the following exercise before you go to sleep tonight.

Write out how you feel about the work you did on your items list between meals today. Was it easy? Fun? A chore? Did you feel like you "won" with any of them? Congratulate yourself for what you accomplished.

20. As you fall asleep tonight, reflect on the experience of your naturally thin day. Congratulate yourself for letting your naturally thin person be in control as much as possible.

WHAT ABOUT TOMORROW?

Now that you've found out first-hand what being "naturally thin" is like, even for a day, it will be easier for you to let go of your old patterns of eating (and *over*eating). Your awareness of the food you eat should increase; it should get easier and easier to disconnect the eating machine and truly enjoy each bite of food you eat.

What you did on your special, first naturally thin day is give yourself a blueprint to follow in the days ahead—and when you look at that in terms of what Dr. Helmstetter has to say about programming, it makes a lot of sense to start giving yourself the program pictures of how *you* look as you begin to live the naturally thin life that is in front of you.

* * * * *

The techniques Dr. Schwartz has outlined for you in this section can be fun—but their real purpose is to help you begin to think and live in a naturally thin way. Even these simple "naturally thin" steps will give you an idea of the kinds of actions you can take—and benefit from—while you practice your Self-Talk.

Now it's time to start putting it all together—and start practicing what we have learned.

Part IV
Putting It All Together

Chapter Twenty-Two

20 Key Questions About Self-Talk For Weight-Loss

Will Self-Talk work for you? If you want to try it, what should you do first? What if you're already on a weight-loss program; should you consider dropping it and trying Self-Talk instead? How long will it take before you notice a difference?

A CHECKLIST OF KEY INFORMATION

What follows are the answers to these and other frequently asked questions about Self-Talk for weight-loss.

1. Does Self-Talk work better for some people than for others?

It is true that virtually anyone can succeed at weight control by using the right Self-Talk. But that doesn't mean everyone will use it the same way, or have the same motivation to begin with.

Some people are better at Self-Talk than others.

That's because some people are ready for it, while others don't want to make any real commitment to change. And because enough Self-Talk always creates change, people who are not ready to make a change will stop using Self-Talk before the long-term improvements begin.

Losing weight permanently, *looking different, becoming healthier,* being *more confident* and *more in control, creating new attitudes*—those changes create some real responsibilities. And in no way to their discredit, some people are not ready for those changes, even if the changes are all positive.

Most other people, however, look *forward* to getting in control. The self-esteem you start feeling when you use Self-Talk is a marvelous experience. Then, too, there are the *other* benefits.

Even the Self-Talk you use just for weight will not stop at just helping you with your weight. It goes beyond that. One man who had listened to Self-Talk to lose 50 pounds called me one day to report what was happening in his life. "My marriage is working better, my job is going great, and my family is getting along better than ever," he said, "and I'm happier than I've ever been." But then he added, sounding a little disappointed, "But I haven't lost all the weight yet. What's wrong?"

That man was doing fine. He just didn't know it yet. The other improvements he was making in his life were so pronounced that they overshadowed the progress he *was* making with his weight.

2. *Is Self-Talk more than a weight-loss program?*

You can't really call Self-Talk a "weight-loss" program, because Self-Talk doesn't just deal with weight. Since

Self-Talk helps you change any area of programs that could be working against you, its coverage is broader than any weight-reduction or maintenance program.

However, Self-Talk also works with weight because it deals with the programs that caused the weight in the first place. When you replace your need to eat beyond what is healthy for you, with different programs that take the need away, many people move from struggling with their weight to a more natural and healthier weight that can be maintained for a lifetime.

ADD SELF-TALK TO ANY WEIGHT PROGRAM YOU ARE USING NOW

Because old programming is *always* a part of the cause of any long-term weight problem, we recommend you add Self-Talk to any good weight-loss or weight-maintenance plan you are now using. If your current weight and fitness program is a good one—that is, if it is working for you—if you add Self-Talk, it will work even better.

3. Can you change your old programs just by being aware of them, or by concentrating on them?

The answer is no, you can't. Neurologically, the more you focus on your old programs, the more you *strengthen* them. Just trying to think about changing old programs not only doesn't work; it can work against you. Self-Talk gives you new programs to focus on while the other, older, harmful programs are weakened as you stop using them entirely.

4. Do you have to go back and "work through" old programs before you can replace them with new programs?

There is a danger in spending too much time going back over past negative programs. The more you *review* them, the more you *renew* them.

Although some forms of therapy require a regressive look at previous experiences, *too much introspection*—as psychologist William James pointed out—*always leads to neurosis.* That is to say, too much looking back can open up old program files that would be better left alone.

Barring the need for professional therapy for some appropriate reason (when in doubt, get help!), it is better to work on creating healthy new programs than revitalizing negative programs from the past. Instead of bringing old programs to life by *reliving* them, reduce their strength by *replacing* them.

5. What if you don't know which of your old programs are causing the weight?

Again, it is better to create healthy new programs than to try to dig up old ones. Remember, too, that Self-Talk is not some form of self-therapy. It is simply the very natural process of giving yourself new programs to follow and then following them. If, for example, your self-esteem is low, and the low self-esteem is causing you to have a weight problem, spend your time building better self-esteem.

If you're not sure which old programs are causing the

weight problem, *don't worry about trying to find out*.
Just get on a solid, comprehensive program of Self-Talk,
and the old programs will take care of themselves. You
can't move forward in life if you're always looking in
your rear-view mirror. If you focus too much on your
past, you have little time and energy left for your present and your future. Let the old programs go. You're
through with them, and you won't be needing them any
longer. The healthiest people are those who focus on
what is working today, and on the goals they want to
reach tomorrow.

6. *Why is Self-Talk always phrased in the present
tense?*

Self-Talk phrases are specific directions to your conscious and your subconscious mind. It is important to
give your subconscious the most complete directions
possible. The more complete the direction, the clearer it
will be.

For that reason, Self-Talk is stated in the present
tense—such as, *"I eat only those things that are healthy
for me."* If you were to say, "I am *going to* eat only those
things that are healthy for me," your subconscious reads
that at face value—just like you stated it. The words
"going to" imply a future event, something that will be
put off until a later time. And as we all know, tomorrow
never comes.

So instead of telling yourself, "This is the way I choose
to be," you would actually be giving yourself the subconscious directive that says, *"I'm not really ready yet.
Maybe I'll eat right some other time."*

Self-Talk is always stated in its most *complete* form—
which is always the present tense. When you give your

programming center a *completed* picture of "you"—how you choose to be in the future—then that is the kind of finished picture that gives the clearest possible directions to your subconscious mind. It is a message that says, *"This is a picture of me the way I choose to be. Now, go to work on it."*

7. Will Self-Talk work if you want to lose a lot of weight?

If you practice and use Self-Talk correctly, which includes staying with it and letting it work, Self-Talk can help you reach any practical weight goal you set.

8. What if you only want to lose a few pounds?

Self-Talk will also help you lose even a few pounds, if that is your goal. Once the healthier new Self-Talk programs start to get in control, the Self-Talk will help you reach *your* goal—any goal—providing the goal itself is healthy and realistic.

9. How long do you have to keep using Self-Talk?

If you really *learn* the new Self-Talk, and stay with it long enough for the new programs to strongly take hold, those new programs will be with you for as long as you live—providing, of course, that you don't once again replace *them* with something else.

To get that whole process started, you should plan on a "start-up" period of at least two to three months. That's no time at all, considering what you will be busy doing for your future in the process. Remember, Self-Talk isn't a temporary diet plan that you use for a while and then give up on; it is a very natural and healthy way of life.

If you choose to listen to Self-Talk Cassettes, you will probably *want* to continue to listen; many people make listening to Self-Talk a permanent part of their lives.

The key here is that once you've reached your healthy weight, it is not necessary to continue listening to the tapes about weight-loss, or using the other Self-Talk techniques to focus on your weight—except during those times that you need extra determination. You can move on to other subjects you want to work on.

10. How long has Self-Talk been practiced?

Self-Talk was first introduced in the United States in its earliest form in the 1970's, by Olympic athletes from Eastern Europe. The concept was also used by NASA astronauts and by commercial airline pilots, both of whom have to be able to make immediate and accurate choices under life-threatening conditions.

The first Self-Talk tapes for the general public, and for weight-loss, were produced in the early 1980's, and have been published continuously since that time. It is estimated that more than two million Self-Talk Cassettes have been produced since their inception.

I have written six previous books on the subject of Self-Talk. The first of these, *What To Say When You Talk To Your Self*, was published in 1986, and was the first popular introduction of the Self-Talk concept to the general public. English and foreign language translations of *What To Say. . .* and the other Self-Talk books are now published in more than 64 countries worldwide.

11. *In what other ways is Self-Talk currently being used?*

The Self-Talk for weight-loss techniques that are discussed in this book are used by many thousands of individuals, along with their use in weight clinics and as an integral part of weight control programs throughout the United States. The concepts are also recommended and prescribed by medical doctors for their patients who are experiencing problems with weight control.

Self-Talk is also used by professional counselors, therapists, psychologists and psychiatrists, to help their clients and patients with many areas of self-esteem and self-reliance, and in individualized therapy and counseling programs.

Self-Talk is taught and used in many other areas, including schools and preschools; churches; businesses; in hospitals, clinics and throughout the health-care fields; in sales organizations; self-help groups; motivational training programs; self-esteem programs; 12-step and similar recovery programs; prisons; in amateur, professional and Olympic athletic programs; in network marketing organizations; and by individuals in many areas of their lives.

12. *Is it necessary to listen to tapes to benefit from Self-Talk?*

You do not have to listen to the Self-Talk on tapes to benefit from Self-Talk, but it is clear that it helps.

The best way to look at this is to compare Self-Talk to a foreign language that you want to learn. There are many ways to learn a new language, but these days the best way is to listen to tapes. The tapes are simply the best way to *naturally* learn the new language, it doesn't take any extra time if you listen while you're doing something else, and it's easy to do.

Practicing the Self-Talk techniques I have outlined will definitely help you, even if you don't listen to tapes. But my objective is to present all of the most helpful reprogramming tools Self-Talk has to offer, and listening to Self-Talk on tapes is among the most frequently used of those tools.

13. What if you don't "believe" the new Self-Talk when you're hearing it or using it?

Perhaps the greatest bonus of practicing Self-Talk is that neurologically, you don't *have* to believe it when you first hear it. The part of the brain that is storing the new programs doesn't care whether we consciously believe them or not; it stores them anyway. What matters most is which program ends up being stronger, chemically and electrically in the brain. The more the same new program is repeated, the stronger it will become.

So a program or a message about you that sounds "impossible" when you first hear it, starts to sound more and more plausible the more times that same message is repeated. In time, that new program becomes the stronger program pathway in the brain. It then gets acted on, and in time, it becomes "fact." So even though you didn't believe it at first, the program ends up being there, and it becomes as real to you as anything else that is "true" about you.

14. How can you use Self-Talk to help someone else with a weight problem (or with some other problem)?

What can you do for someone else—someone who lives with you, or someone else you care about—who has a problem, and you want to help?

If that person *wants* your help, then sharing what you know about Self-Talk is a good place to start. By itself, though, that won't change anything. If that person really wants to make a change, then it will be up to him or her to practice using Self-Talk just like you would use it. Many people have helped someone else in just that way, so you may want to try introducing the person you want to help to Self-Talk.

But what if you want to help other people change their self-talk, and they are unwilling to work at it?

First of all, don't try to force the Self-Talk concept on them. That won't help, and it will only make the person more resistant to your help. What many people have had success with in similar situations is to play their own Self-Talk tapes quietly in the background each day, where the other person can hear them. The tapes should be played in the *background* anyway, and their new Self-Talk messages *will* be getting through to the other person as long as the tapes can be heard. But don't make an issue of telling that person he or she *ought* to listen; just let the tapes do what they are designed to do, quietly and naturally creating new programs both for you and for the other people you care about.

I receive many letters from people who started using Self-Talk for themselves, and then other family members in the household started doing better *without even trying to*. A lot of parents, as an example, have found that their children were getting along better at home and doing better at school, all because the parents were listening to Self-Talk to help them fix something in their own lives. The children were the beneficiaries of the parents' new Self-Talk.

The important point in this is that a person doesn't have to *try* to "listen" to the Self-Talk tapes or focus on them consciously for the Self-Talk to work. The result is that if you want to help someone else, you can; there is something you can do.

15. If you change your Self-Talk, can you still eat anything you want?

I am sometimes surprised by the number of people who have asked me if they get to eat as much as they want if they use Self-Talk at the same time.

I can understand the hopefulness in that question. But I suspect they know better. Self-Talk isn't capable of removing calories or fat grams from food; it is intended, rather, to make it *easier* and more *natural* to eat the right foods and in the right amount.

That would mean that in time, as the Self-Talk changes how you look at food (and other things in your life), you end up *not wanting* something that is un-healthy for you. The result is you no longer want to eat more than you should. The bottom line is: *of course* you still have to follow the "rules" of healthy eating and moderate exercise in order to lose weight—but the right program of Self-Talk deals with the motivation and programming changes you need in order to stick with the process and make it work for you.

16. Will Self-Talk improve your self-esteem?

Yes. It is the building of self-esteem that is the greatest benefit of practicing Self-Talk. Every time you use the right kind of Self-Talk, you build self-esteem. Every time your self-esteem improves, your own Self-Talk gets better. When your Self-Talk gets better, your self-esteem goes up another notch, and so on and so on. And so begins the positive cycle of building *much* stronger self-esteem and getting in control of your life.

The right Self-Talk is the *key* to self-esteem. In fact, your self-esteem today is literally the result of the programs you have right now. Your self-esteem *tomorrow* and in the future will be the direct result of the programs you create next—and Self-Talk is the most effective method for creating the right new programs.

COULD MOST WEIGHT PROBLEMS BE THE RESULT OF *LOW* SELF-ESTEEM?

Most behavioral researchers who understand the neurological and chemical side of programming would answer "yes" to that question.

Your internal image of who you are, what you are capable of doing, the strengths you have, and the choices you make—that image is the result of the self-esteem programs you carry with you right now.

Those same programs end up deciding what you eat; how much you eat and how often; how much exercise you get; and everything else you do that results in what you weigh and how you look. You end up becoming the *result* of the strongest pictures of yourself that you carry in your mind.

When you improve your self-esteem, you will, in time,

improve everything else about you. That's how programming works. And that's very good news, because if you want to improve your self-esteem, you can. Self-Talk is one of the best ways we have ever found of doing that.

17. Can Self-Talk help your children?

Self-Talk *can* help children, and in many more ways than just controlling weight. If you consider the fact that the programs our children receive are literally setting up who they are, *right now,* and what they will do *every day,* there may be nothing more important we can give our children than the right programs of Self-Talk.

Children learn to use Self-Talk in much the same way that adults learn it, although they usually learn the new Self-Talk faster than we do, since they have fewer old programs to undo, and they take to tapes very naturally. There are also Self-Talk tapes that are specially written and recorded just for children and for young people.

DON'T FOCUS ON THE WEIGHT— FOCUS ON THE SELF-ESTEEM

When you want to help a child or a young person *specifically* with Self-Talk for weight-loss, it is important to use the Self-Talk to build *self-esteem*, but *avoid focusing on the "weight" as a problem*. Unless there is a physical, medical reason for the child's weight problem, the basis of the problem will *always* be found in his or her self-esteem, and that is the area you should focus on. The rule is: get away from the subject of "weight", and *immediately* start using Self-Talk that builds self-esteem.

18. What should you do if it's hard to get started?

Over a period of several years, I have conducted hundreds of Self-Talk seminars, many of them for weight-loss. I have noticed a curious thing about the people who attend the seminars. When the subject of the Self-Talk seminar is about general "success," almost all of the people who attend show up on time. But when the seminar is about weight-loss, many of the people show up late—and some of them not at all.

And I'm not the only individual who has observed the high percentage of people who procrastinate about weight control. The phenomenon is universal.

In the hundreds of weight-control programs he has conducted throughout the country, Dr. Schwartz, too, has experienced the exact same pattern: if the seminar session was about weight control, some people would inevitably put it off until the last possible moment. Dr. Schwartz also concluded that many of the people who wanted to be there never showed up.

The conclusion is clear that *doing* something about weight is an easy thing to put off. The people who attended the weight-loss seminars were not forced to be there. They decided on their own to attend, and they went there of their own free will. And yet, they showed up at the seminar as late as they could, delaying the inevitable commitment as long as they possibly could.

But don't be discouraged if you fall into the category of those who procrastinate about weight control. Putting off "taking it off" is a common problem. And it is a problem that is created entirely by old programs that *want* to stop you from changing them! If you have any feelings that tell you the Self-Talk techniques won't work for you, or that you should wait for some other time to start, then I recommend that you begin using the techniques *immediately*.

The sooner you begin, the quicker you will start to replace the old programs that are trying to stop you from reaching your weight-loss goals.

19. Is it best to start slowly, or all at once?

It's best to practice as many of the Self-Talk techniques as you can—*especially* when you are getting started. Go ahead, let yourself experience what it feels like to *take control*—not just control of your weight, but of everything about you. Take an active and energetic role in your success! Start "turning on" the Self-Talk in every way you can. The more of yourself you put into it, the better you will do.

20. If you learn Self-Talk, are you certain to get in control of your weight?

If you practice Self-Talk—if you follow the techniques while following the other basic rules of losing weight—and if you stay with it, it will work.

We know this for certain: if you consume fewer calories and less fat than your body requires to operate, you will lose weight. And if you don't, you won't. There is nothing known to modern medicine, chemistry, or physics that will change that. It is an unbreakable physical law.

Here are some other basic rules to follow:

❏ Avoid fad diets of *any kind*. Eat the right kind of foods, and make sure you get the nutrition you need. If you want to lose weight, reduce your fat intake to less than your body burns, and eat only when your *body* is hungry.

❏ Engage only in sensible, moderate exercise. Avoid trying *any* unusual or extreme exercise program as a way to lose weight. For long-term weight maintenance, don't even start an exercise program that you would not enjoy still being on at least five or ten years from now.

❏ Set realistic weight goals and review them frequently, until each goal is met. (See Chapter 23, Self-Talk And Setting Goals.)

❏ Begin immediately practicing the Self-Talk techniques.

It is this fourth rule, practicing your Self-Talk, that will help you follow the other three rules—*and make them work*. That's how Self-Talk helps you lose weight, and keep it off. It is the Self-Talk that will help you build your self-esteem and your self-confidence, help you make better choices, and help you stick to them. And it is the Self-Talk that gives you a way to override the old programs that caused the problem in the first place.

If you learn Self-Talk, you will be giving yourself an advantage nothing else we know of can give you. If you use the new Self-Talk—if you learn it, practice it, and make it a part of your life—you will win.

Chapter Twenty-Three
Self-Talk And Setting Goals

Out of every hundred people you might meet, how many of them would you guess set goals and write them down?

Most estimates put the answer at less than 5%. I believe the actual number is even lower—less than three out of a hundred people actually *set* goals regularly, write them down, review them, and follow a preset plan to reach them. That has always seemed surprising when you consider that *no one* seems to disagree with the *idea* of setting goals. It is one of those things everyone agrees they ought to do, even if they haven't gotten around to it yet.

Another of the immutable laws of weight control is this:

If you want to maintain or control your weight permanently, you must set goals.

I now believe there is no exception to that rule. If you want to get in control and stay in control of your weight for a long period of time, and you do not practice setting goals, you will never be completely in control. There may be some achievers who set goals rather casually, or naturally—that is, they don't focus on the goals deliberately and write them down—but they are the rare exceptions.

I have been studying people engaged in the art of achieving success now for more than twenty-five years and I have yet to find a single truly and completely "successful" individual who did not set goals. I would even take the rule I stated above, one step further: Goal-setting in any successful endeavor is essential; goal-setting in weight control is *crucial*.

The reason most people don't set goals properly is because they don't really know how to. There were few classes on goal-setting offered in school. That is in spite of the fact that the techniques of good goal-setting are among the simplest techniques ever taught. They are easy to learn, easy to apply, and easy to keep up with. There's no good reason at all not to use them, except for the fact that setting goals, too, is a habit—one that we either have learned or we haven't. Fortunately, that is a problem we can fix.

If you do not currently set specific goals, if you do not write them down, and follow them faithfully, the practice of setting goals in the right way could be, by itself, the turning point in your success with weight control.

YOU *CAN* SET GOALS AND GET THEM RIGHT

Some people are not fair with themselves. They say they are going to do something—in this case, reach and maintain some desired weight—but they never quite do it. They either set their intentions too low or their expectations too high.

One of the skills you will develop when you consistently set and follow well-planned goals—*while* you are practicing Self-Talk—is the ability to set your expectations at a realistic level. When it comes to setting weight goals the word "realistic" means the weight you really *are* going to reach (or maintain) by the date you set. That doesn't mean you'll always hit your target; it means the target you set is always a target you *could* hit if you did all the right things.

The reason it is important that your written goals be realistic is that each time you fail to reach one of your planned targets, you give yourself another program that says, "*I fail when I set goals.*" (How's *that* for bad programming?) So if you write down a goal that is unrealistic, each day that goes by your mind is repeating that same bad program to you again and again, *knowing* you won't be able to reach your goal.

In the same way, every time you set a realistic goal and give yourself an honest chance of *reaching* it, you also give yourself a repeated program that says, "*When I set goals I reach them!*"

The rule to follow is simple: Always set the most realistic goal possible. If your goal is to reach a weight that is too low, that weight will be impossible to reach—or maintain—and you will set up a pattern of failure.

On the other hand, if your goal is too easy and asks nothing of you, it is impossible to become fully committed, and no personal excitement or enthusiasm enters your goal plan. If you don't expect enough of yourself, you will never give yourself the chance to learn how capable you really are. The prudent choice is to always set goals that are practical and realistic—goals that expect the best of yourself.

A NEW LOOK AT YOUR PERSONAL GOALS

In the following goal-setting steps you'll be asked to write down some very specific goals. Give yourself some time. Think them over. Be honest and be practical. And above all, make the choice to believe in yourself and in your ability to reach each of them.

The basics of goal-setting have been taught for years. More recently, however, we've learned more about how the brain processes and stores goals, so the newer techniques have gotten easier and they are more effective. The reason is that a combination of the right goals—*and* the right Self-Talk—used *together*, make the best goal-setting methods work better.

The goals you set when you're using Self-Talk will almost always be different than the goals you had set before. Self-Talk shows you a picture of what you *can* accomplish, and it overrides old programs that tell you you're not good enough. So the pictures of your future you'll be seeing now—or after practicing Self-Talk—could be very different pictures from those you've seen in the past.

To make sure you're getting the *right* mental pictures of yourself when you begin setting your new goals, I recommend reading or rereading the Self-Talk scripts from the previous chapters. If you're going to listen to Self-Talk on tapes, listen to one of the tapes just before you sit down to work on your goal plan.

Even just *reading* the scripts by themselves will give you a stronger picture of you, and it will be easier to see yourself accomplishing the goals you are setting. And *that* will help you set more realistic goals to begin with.

THREE SIMPLE, PRACTICAL GOALS

The following steps are designed to be used along with the Self-Talk techniques I have outlined in the preceding chapters. Now that you have a clear picture of how the Self-Talk works and how it can help you, it's time to begin by setting your new goals.

☐ *Choose your most natural desired weight and write it down.*

Think about this one for a while. What is the most natural weight you would like to maintain? Make sure you don't overstate the weight and don't understate it. What weight would really be the healthiest for you?

Be practical, but don't sell yourself short either. If the weight is one you haven't reached yet, could you realistically reach it? If food or eating were *not* a problem, could you do it? And most important, would that weight be a natural, healthy weight for you?

What is that number?

Whatever that final number is for you, write it down in the blank provided on the sample Personal Goal Plan at the end of this chapter. If you choose not to write in the book, make a photo-copy of the Goal Plan and fill in the blanks on your copy.

Note: Since this is not a book about "diets," we have refrained from restating any of the commonly recommended foods or quantities that many diet programs suggest. You should note, however, that most current nutritional experts agree with the recommendation that losing one pound of fat per week is a sensible goal. Dr. Schwartz gives the example of carrying four sticks of margarine around for a week. Taking *off* one pound of fat a week for one year equals fifty-two pounds less fat.

Your own goal should always be based on your doctor's advice, good nutrition and common sense.

❐ *Choose the weight you want to weigh at the end of this month.*

This will be your first "near-term" goal. It asks you to think about what you are actually going to weigh on the last day of the current month. Even if that date is only three or four days from now, decide what you will weigh on that date and write it in the blank provided on the Personal Goal Plan I've outlined for you.

❐ *Write out the three most important "action steps" you will take to help you reach your month-end goal.*

An example of one woman's goal-plan list included follow-up steps such as:

1. *Eat no more than 30 grams of fat in any one day.*

2. *Practice or listen to Self-Talk each morning, at meal-time, and before bed each night.*

3. *Take a twenty minute morning walk at least four times a week.*

For *your* goal plan, write down any action step you believe will help you reach your first goal. Anything that will help you can be written down, but make sure whatever action steps you select are steps you *will* do. If it's a "maybe" idea, something that is too hard to do, too hard to remember to do, or something that is too easy to put off until another day, don't write it down.

First, on a separate sheet of paper (not in your goal plan), write down every action step idea you can think of. Then, once you have gone through your list several times, select your three best action steps and write *those* steps in your Personal Goal Plan.

In your goal plan, write down *only* those action steps you're really going to follow up on. Once again, use the "simple and easy" rule. If it isn't simple and easy *for you* to do, don't write it down in the first place.

Your action steps should be those steps that work for *you*. To give you ideas, here are some other examples of action steps other people have written down and used successfully:

Keep a fat gram log, and fill it out before every meal.

Read at least one book on low-fat cooking this month.

Take down the "overweight" pictures from the refrigerator door and put up pictures of me when I was thin.

Ask Paul (husband) to encourage me, especially when I'm doing well.

Get a new "doctor's scale."

Plan all of my meals (3) each day. Make sure they help me reach my goal plan for this month.

Buy gold stars at the office supply and give myself an award on my weight chart every night I've stayed with it.

Replace red meat with fish or chicken. No oil or butter.

Don't put extra salt on anything.

Read my goal plan and my action steps every morning and every night.

Practice thinking like a naturally thin person every time I go shopping.

Use the Situational Self-Talk I'm practicing every time I sit down to eat.

Throw out my oversized clothes.

As you can see, some of the action steps are just good habits for *any* health-conscious person to follow. Other action steps are shorter-term "boosts" to help you get started.

Whatever you believe will work for you, think about it, write it down, and then select your three best ideas from your list and write them in the appropriate place in your Personal Goal Plan below.

Adding the right action steps to your goal plan is important. People who do not think about and write down what they're going to do to make their plan work, seldom reach their goal. The secret to setting goals isn't just the goal itself; it's the little things you do each day that actually get you there. And in this step, taking the time to think about those first steps you're going to take will begin to help you practice "thinking" achievement.

When you decide on something you want, and then write down specific steps to help you get it, you are focusing on the achievement. The more you focus, the more you see yourself having reached your goal, the more of your brain's natural programming energy will be applied to the task. So writing action steps doesn't just help you decide what you're going to do next; it also *programs* the picture of accomplishment into your brain.

☐ *Write down the weight you choose to be at—exactly one year from now.*

Use the same "reality" criteria for setting your one-year goal as you use for each of your monthly goals. Get a clear picture of where you want your weight and fitness to be, and write down your weight goal in the goal plan. (You may include your other physical measurements, but those are optional.) Whatever you write down in your plan will help determine what you do for the next 12 months.

☐ *Write out the six most important "action steps" that you will follow to reach your one-year goal.*

Just as you did earlier for your end-of-the-month goal, make a separate list—as many ideas as you can write down—of the action steps you could take to help you reach your goal. Then select the best *six* of these and write them down in your goal plan.

HOW YOU WANT TO BE *FIVE YEARS* FROM NOW WILL TELL YOU WHAT TO DO TODAY

Goals like these have a way of making themselves

come true—almost as though they have an energy and a power of their own. A good example of this is a friend of mine who told me he wanted to show me his goal cards. He proudly took out a pack of about a dozen 5X8 index cards with goals, dates, and action steps clearly written out on each of them. My friend then read through the cards, reading only the goal statement on the top of each. When he got through, it was clear that my friend had just read me a detailed picture, not of what he wanted to achieve, but rather, where he was in his life already. The statements on the cards and his life at the moment were a perfect match.

"Those don't sound like goals," I told my friend. "They sound more like your biography." And indeed the list of accomplishments the cards outlined did sound a lot like the attributes I might list for my friend if I were introducing him to an audience.

"That's just it!" my friend said happily. "That's exactly what *I* thought as I read these cards to myself when I found them this morning. I was going through some old things in my desk and I recognized what they were. *I haven't seen these goal cards for over five years,*" my friend said. "And everything I wrote down on them has come true!"

My favorite expression about goal-setting is the popular phrase: "Be careful what you want . . . you'll probably get it." And I would add to that phrase, "If you *write it down*, it will almost *certainly* happen." The fact is, the simple step of writing your goals down on paper is the one most important step you can take in the setting of goals.

❏ *Write down the weight you choose to be — exactly five years from now.*

231

Wave your wand. Imagine yourself being exactly how you'd *like* to be five years from now. If you do what you already know you should do to keep yourself in the healthiest physical condition, how much will you weigh at the end of five years?

This goal is critical. This is the goal that will set the "master" program in place for all of your other health and fitness goals to follow. This is the kind of goal that changes the choices that change your life.

☐ *Write out a complete physical description of you—as you plan to be—five years from now.*

Imagine that you had a special kind of camera that could take a picture of you today, but when you saw the print it would be a picture of you as you will look exactly five years from now. To complete this step in your goal plan, all you have to do is describe *that* photograph.

How do you look? How much do you weigh? If measurements are important to you, what are yours? How is your general physical health? What color is your hair? How well do you take care of yourself? What do you do to exercise? How much exercise do you get? How do you feel? Is weight a problem to you now? What kinds of things do you like to eat? What kinds of habits do you have? Are you happy? Are you in control of your life?

Answer each of those questions as though you were describing you as you would *most like to be* five years from right now. Be realistic, be practical about this, but also give yourself a chance to see yourself at your best.

☐ *Write down the six most important "action steps" you will take to help you reach your five-year goal.*

This final goal, and the six action steps that go with it, could be the most important goal you will ever set. *This* goal stands above all of the other goals that went before it. Because it is this goal—your own prediction about yourself and how you choose to be—that, if it is strong enough, will end up governing everything else you do from here on out. And it will be from this goal, more than any other goals you set, that the "magic" will come.

WHAT IS THE "MAGIC" THAT MAKES GOALS COME TRUE?

During my study of more than fifty years of self-help concepts, this notion of the almost "*magical*" quality of goal-setting has come up time and time again.

There have been many books written which have attested to some mystical quality of strong desires which are transmuted into clearly-defined goals—and which, in turn, take on an almost spiritual power that turns them into reality. And I would have to say that I, too, have witnessed this phenomenon take place in many people's lives and even in my own life. When it happens, it *does* appear to be magical, and incredibly powerful.

But where does that power to transform goals into reality really come from? Does it come from some *spiritual* source as many say it does? It certainly seems to.

Does it come from intense *desire,* secretly filling the goal itself with limitless energy, as others have suggested? That could be. Desire does seem to help.

Does the goal lift itself to life on the wings of *faith,* as others have told us? There is no doubt that faith can move the mountains they say it does.

But I would suggest that when a goal turns from a simple idea into a living reality, its true pathway to achievement comes from something far less mystical.

Consider what we now know about programs in the human brain: Imagine for a moment that your "goal" is a new directive that you "type" into your subconscious mind. Imagine also that this new directive, this goal, is typed in very clearly, and it includes precise action steps and a clear picture of the final outcome.

Now put a program like that into action neurologically—*chemically and electrically*—by imprinting it into the human brain! Record it so deeply and so strongly in the program pathways of the brain that it begins to duplicate and repeat its message *again and again*, changing a small choice here, an action there, and then dozens of those small choices and actions, and then *thousands* of them, relentlessly following the same strong program path again and again, growing chemically stronger with each repeated use of that same powerful program.

Weeks and months go by, and while life moves on around it, that program never sleeps. In time that goal—now a powerful new program in the brain—begins to override *old* program paths, and the old paths begin to lose their energy and give way, no longer as strong as the mighty new program that is replacing them. And because this new program is now stronger than all the others, it reigns supreme, overpowering, relentless, and unstoppable.

And one day, some time later after months or a year or more has gone by, you look around you, almost surprised by what has happened: your goal has come to life.

You have *changed*, and your world has changed.

That quiet goal, written simply in a goal plan and cared for properly, began its journey to life in the program paths of your brain. And once there, nurtured and allowed to grow, it created a chain of events—*a network of neurological patterns*—so strong and pervasive, that *nothing* could slow it or stop it.

That is what turns a goal into reality. And *that* is the power of programs in action.

Whatever goals you write in your plan, you can afford to take them very seriously. Write them down. Follow them up with the right steps of action. Nurture your goals. Care for them like you would care for the very essence of yourself. Then add faith, fill them with spirit, and give to them all of the desire you feel in your heart.

Do that, and one day you may well look back at the day you first set those goals, and it will seem as though your goals have a magic of their own. It won't have been magic at all, of course. Even if other people think you have changed your looks or your life by some divine gift of good fortune, you and I will know the truth. We will know that the "magic" was *you*.

YOUR PERSONAL GOAL PLAN

Complete the goal plan on the next three pages. (Make photocopies as necessary.) After you have completed all the information in the goal plan, follow these five steps:

1. For the next 30 days, read your goal plan once a day.

2. On the first day of next month, reset your next "end-of-the-month" goal. Continue to reset your monthly

goal on the first day of each month.

3. After the first 30 days, read your goal plan a *minimum* of once each week for 6 months.

4. After 6 months, read your goal plan a *minimum* of once every month.

5. On the first day of each month (or once every 30 days) adjust your goal plan as appropriate.

MY PERSONAL GOAL PLAN

A. The healthiest weight for me to be is: _____.

B. My desired weight I plan to weigh on the last day of this month is _____ pounds. Today's date is _____.

The three Action Steps I will take to achieve my monthly goal are:

1. _____
_____

2. _____
_____

3. _____
_____

C. The desired weight I plan to weigh on (date)_____, one year from today, is_____ pounds.

The six Action Steps I will take to achieve my one-year goal are:

1. _____
_____

2. _____
_____

3. _____

_____

4. _____

_____

5. _____

_____

6. _____

_____

D. *The desired weight I plan to weigh on (date)_____,
five years from today, is____ pounds.*

   *The six Action Steps I will take to achieve my five-year
goal are:*

1. _____

_____

2. _____

_____

3. _____

_____

4. _____

_____

5. _____
   _____

6. _____
   _____

E. The following is a description of me as I choose to be five years from today:

_____
_____
_____
_____
_____
_____
_____
_____
_____
_____
_____
_____
_____

*Your signature*_____

*Today's date*_____.

Chapter Twenty-Four

The Three Stages Of Self-Talk : You've Got A Lot To Look Forward To

When you start using Self-Talk, you have a lot to look forward to. What comes next could be very exciting for you.

Self-Talk *still* continues to surprise me. Even after working with Self-Talk for many years, I am still amazed at the vastness of its effect on our lives.

Due to my own conservative nature, I have always underplayed Self-Talk's greatest successes. I don't often talk about the fifteen and sixteen-year-old kids who have gotten off drugs because of Self-Talk. I am often hesitant to mention the men and women who have moved from alcoholism to freedom from drink because they learned to change their programs with Self-Talk.

When I am asked by the host of a radio or television program during an interview, to share the success stories, I never mention the man who lost the 140 pounds or the woman who lost 85. I have seldom told the stories of Self-Talk saving people's lives and bringing them from near-suicide to being more alive than ever. I have refused to talk even about my own children and grandchildren, and how their lives have become testaments to the value of exceptional self-esteem.

I have resisted the inclination to shower my readers with grand promises of unlimited futures, knowing that we are given too many of these promises already.

But I mention these pictures of Self-Talk working in people's lives, now, because it is important that you know what to expect. You should know what could be ahead for you if you decide to make the simple choice to do everything you can to bring Self-Talk into your life, now.

If you begin practicing the techniques I am recommending to you in this book, and if you stay with them, you can be certain you will begin to create some very positive benefits in your life. There is no question at all about that. If you practice the techniques—if you *use* it—Self-Talk *will* help.

THE FIRST STAGE OF SELF-TALK— AWARENESS, PRACTICE, AND NEW MOTIVATION

During the years we have studied the results Self-Talk is creating, we have learned that Self-Talk works in three fairly distinct stages. The first stage is made up of a combination of *awareness*, *practice*, and *new motivation*.

1. *Awareness*

This phase is very likely happening for you already,

even if this is your first introduction to Self-Talk. At the *awareness* level, you start to think about Self-Talk in general, and programming, and to some extent, about using the new Self-Talk as a possible replacement for the old.

This is the phase in which we start to listen to our own self-talk as it is now, and also when we start to listen to what other people are saying—we start to notice *their* self-talk, too. At this level, some people become *very* aware of their old self-talk (and their old programs) and they give it a lot of thought. They may think about some of their strongest programs and where they came from. Most people now begin to come up with a program or two—or a *lot* of them—they would like to change.

It is during this phase that some people experience a "breakthrough" of sorts; they are suddenly confronted with the recognition that perhaps *everything* they have ever done might be the result of programs. That recognition often leads to the further awareness that everyone around them is just responding to their *own* programs—and an early result is that they start to look at other people differently.

A TIME TO MAKE NEW DECISIONS

It is in the first *awareness* phase that you begin to make some decisions. It is an *exciting* time! Imagine the doors that begin to open up in front of you when you consider getting rid of the old programs that put the doors there in the first place!

Do you want to weigh less? Would you like to lose weight more easily? Imagine once getting rid of the weight, being able to keep it off without having to worry about it coming back.

Or how about those other areas of your life that could be affected just as positively as your weight? Imagine getting rid of the "negatives," being more in control, knowing what you want and reaching the kind of goals you thought were reserved for someone else. Maybe you would like to make some important improvements in your marriage or in your family, or perhaps in your job or your career.

Or maybe you want to do something more with your life, but you either haven't had the time or you just didn't think it was *possible*.

The biggest problem with dreaming is that we don't do enough of it. One of the earliest programs many of us got was to stop daydreaming and pay attention. We got awfully good at paying attention; we got so good at it that now we get up, go to work, come home, eat, get tired, and go to bed—all the while paying attention to what we have to do just to get by, but never stopping long enough to pay attention to *us*.

IT'S TIME TO DREAM AGAIN!

It's time for you! It *is* time to dream again. It's time to sit down and take a good look at yourself and think about what you really want.

Go ahead. You not only deserve it, you *need* to dream for yourself. What are you doing when you're the happiest—*really* happiest? Where are you? How do you look? What are you wearing? How do you feel? Who are the people you have around you then? What would you do in your spare time? What do you like to do most? What makes you smile? What makes you feel most secure and contented with your life? What are some of the new pictures of *you* your life is putting in front of you when you dream?

Wherever that place is, whatever it is you are doing there, *that* "you" has the right to live in the sunshine of a beautiful and exceptional life. Accepting anything less is nothing more than tired old programs from the past trying to hold you back, unwilling to change, and not wanting to let you stop them.

Don't let them stop you. Stop *them*!

When your awareness of the new Self-Talk begins to show you what lies beyond the looking glass, remember that it isn't magic at all. It's real. It is you, choosing to live—right now—the life you have now, and not waiting for someone, or something, or some other time to stop you.

2. Practice

A woman asked me which of the various Self-Talk techniques I would recommend she practice if she wanted to be absolutely sure she would be successful. My answer was very clear. *Start with all of them.* Try them out. Get familiar with all of them and get to know the ones you like best.

Start right away. Monitor your own current self-talk; listen to it and learn what it says. Practice turning it around and restating it every chance that comes along. If you can, listen to the tapes. Make them as much a part of your day as getting up in the morning. In every way you use it, let the new language of Self-Talk come to life in everything you think and do during the day.

Practice making your new choices with the new Self-Talk always there, already becoming a part of you, inside, making sure you are in complete control of even the smallest choices you make.

Practice using the new Self-Talk at every meal and in between. Give yourself the directions that put *you* in control. Consciously "type" the right programs into your computer every possible chance you get: when you're getting up in the morning, looking in the mirror, choosing the outfit you're going to wear that day, writing down your monthly goal, filling out your weight chart, driving through the fast food restaurant, driving to work, talking to your friends, standing in front of the snack machine, sitting down in a restaurant, shopping for groceries, fixing dinner, at home, during each meal, spending time with your family, laying your head down on your pillow each night, and drifting off into sleep. If you want to succeed, those are the times when you should practice the new Self-Talk.

In most of those instances, it won't take a moment of extra time, it won't ask you to make a sweeping change in your life, and it won't ask you to do anything that is impossible or even too difficult.

CREATING A HABIT YOU WILL WANT TO HOLD ON TO

I have often given gifts of Self-Talk tapes to people who were unsure of themselves, or who otherwise could not have obtained them. In doing so, I have asked the individual to agree with me that they would practice the Self-Talk techniques I outlined for them, with one of those techniques being that they simply play specific Self-Talk tapes that I have recommended, quietly in the background once each morning, when possible during the day, and then just once while they are going to sleep at night.

I have also asked those same individuals, two or three weeks later, if they would be willing to give up practicing any of the Self-Talk techniques, including listening to tapes each day. Not one of them was willing to stop using the techniques or give up the tapes I had given to them.

That is because practicing Self-Talk becomes a habit in itself. The more you do it, the more automatically you do it again. Try practicing exactly the right kind of new Self-Talk the very first thing as you're waking up each morning for three or four weeks without fail. Do the same thing for three weeks during the *rest* of your day as well, and watch what happens.

At the end of just a few short weeks you will not have changed any deep-seated long-term programs. But even after that short period of time, try waking up the very next morning and telling yourself it's going to be a *terrible* day. It will be almost impossible to even say the words. Your own new Self-Talk will have already started to create more good programs just like it, and to fight off the bad programs that had gotten in your way.

THE WOMAN WHO DID NOTHING BUT WAIT

I remember one woman who told me that she was afraid Self-Talk was not going to work for her. "I have waited for three months," she told me, "and I haven't reached my weight goal yet."

"And what have you done to help yourself lose the weight?" I asked her.

"Why, nothing," she said. "I thought the weight was supposed to just go away by itself!"

Obviously her old programs were still letting her kid herself. Even the best, strongest Self-Talk in the world won't tie your hands behind your back at dinner, or write your goals out and read them each morning *for* you. The Self-Talk is there to encourage and help motivate you while you are working at changing old programs—but making the decision to succeed, and then taking action on your goal every chance you get, is still up to you.

Self-Talk doesn't absolve you of taking responsibility for yourself; it does just the opposite. Even practicing Self-Talk to begin with is saying,

"I choose to take responsibility for myself and for every action I take.

I know that my weight control is all up to me, and I choose to take action now.

I do everything I need to do to make sure that I am reaching my goal."

Letting Self-Talk begin to work naturally in your life doesn't mean sitting down and waiting for it to happen. It means *practicing* Self-Talk in an easy and consistent way, while you get used to it—and meanwhile, doing everything *you* can to help it work.

Practice may not make perfect—but practice *does* change programs.

3. *New Motivation*

The first result of the "awareness" and the "practice" of Self-Talk is *new motivation*. Motivation means to be "put into motion." Learning Self-Talk and practicing it literally changes what you do next. Within days of getting started, many people begin looking at their food and looking at mealtime differently. They may not suddenly change all their eating habits, but they notice that *something* is changing their attitudes about eating.

But sitting down to eat is just a small part of what makes up natural lifetime weight control.

How do you choose to spend the rest of your time? How do you feel about yourself today, each day—how is your self-esteem?

Have you written down your goals yet? Are you thinking about reaching your first monthly goal?

Have you spent any time planning what you're going to do a year from now when your first annual milestone is behind you and you're busy opening up the doors to the rest of your life?

Are you beginning to surround yourself with people who have the kind of attitude that will help you succeed?

Are you watching the rest of your Self-Talk and making sure it's the right kind? Are you being organized, getting things done, and getting in control?

All of those kinds of everyday activities and attitudes are *motivated* by your Self-Talk. The new motivation that begins when you practice Self-Talk will give you a boost in areas of your life that seem, at the moment, to have nothing to do with controlling your weight. But it is *exactly* that sort of extra-curricular motivation that makes it easier for you to gain control of everything *else* that controls your weight.

As we have learned, it is not just your "diet, food, eating, and weight" programs that control your weight. Your weight is governed by the programs that control the other facets of your life. During the first stage of Self-Talk, you will begin to experience new motivation in those other areas of your life, as well.

WHAT TO LOOK FOR DURING STAGE ONE

You'll know when the Self-Talk is working. If you are like most of us, several, or possibly all, of the following positive signs of Self-Talk starting to work, will show up during the first days or weeks you are practicing. The more techniques you use—the more you practice—the quicker and more apparently these benefits or effects will start to appear:

1. Your old self-talk will start to be more noticeable.

The more you "listen" for your old programs, the more you'll hear them. The techniques we've suggested help you do this. With some practice, being aware of your old self-talk will come naturally to you.

2. You'll immediately start to notice the "negative" self-talk of others.

You may even find yourself wanting to help other people by helping them edit what they say when their self-talk is "showing." It's a good idea to resist the temptation to correct someone else's self-talk, but it will point out how *aware* of Self-Talk you are starting to become. After a while you'll get used to hearing how "down" some

249

people's self-talk can be. During this stage you may also begin to notice the difference in the self-talk between people who are very successful and people who are not.

Meanwhile, every time you hear someone else using the *wrong* kind of self-talk it will remind you again of the great *new* Self-Talk that *you're* using.

3. If you are setting goals and beginning to work on them, you should notice the first changes in your eating habits.

You probably won't suddenly stop overeating or stop eating all fats the moment you start practicing Self-Talk. Overnight weight-loss is never a permanent solution, and it is not the intent of Self-Talk to start you on another fast or fad.

But if weight-*loss* is a goal of yours, during the first stage of using Self-Talk, you will not only begin to think about your health differently, you will probably start to change your *natural* eating habits. Instead of "dieting," it is quite common for Self-Talkers to begin making important adjustments in what they put on their plates. If you don't already know the healthy "rules" on fat grams, remember to pick up an up-to-date nutrition book to give you the basics.

It is not at all unusual to start correcting eating habits within the first two to three weeks of using Self-Talk. Remember, eating "habits" are just that, *habits*, so it's a good idea to keep in mind that neurologically, in the brain, any new habit you want to create has to be patterned and followed for about three weeks *just to get the process started*.

Since we are talking about making positive changes that you want to stay with for the rest of your life, asking yourself to work for a few weeks to begin to put some new habits into place is not a great investment. If it seems difficult at first, that's just because the new habit programs you are creating are not standing up and walking by themselves yet.

Nurture them. Take care of them. These new habits— these new *programs*—you're creating, will take care of *you* for a lot longer than it took you to create them in the first place.

4. You will notice an increase in your motivation and in your desire to succeed.

The strength of your motivation will be directly related to how much new Self-Talk you are using. If you want to have more energy and more determination—practice or listen to more Self-Talk. That's important, because meanwhile, there could be some old programs trying to stop you:

5. Your old programs will try to tell you that this will not work.

The old programs will do anything they can to convince you to stop. If you hear yourself saying, *"This can't possibly work for me,"* you are hearing your old programs talking. But stay with it. You control them—don't let them convince you to stop.

One woman said of Self-Talk, after hearing it for only a few minutes, "That's too simple. I'd feel silly doing it." If she had changed the word "silly" to the word "different" she would have been more accurate. Yes, you will feel *different* using the new Self-Talk.

You *should* feel different. You're using entirely different programs. If you feel just the same as before, think the same, and do all of the same things you did before, of course you won't feel "silly," or even "different." But then, you won't change any old programs, either.

6. *Other people around you, at home or at work, may try to discourage you.*

Making important changes in your own life can be threatening to people around you. Sometimes their security is based on things *not* changing. So even if they are people who otherwise care about you, they may make comments to you that could be negative or discouraging.

Don't listen to them. Tell yourself the words,

"I no longer live my life based on the negative opinions of others."

"I no longer live my life based on the negative opinions of others."

"I no longer live my life based on the negative opinions of others."

(That is an excellent example of using *Situational* Self-Talk.) If people around you aren't as encouraging as they ought to be, or if they'd like to see you stop before you get started, keep that and a few other well-chosen phrases of Self-Talk around, ready for you to use at a moment's notice! Repeat them to yourself, or say them out loud if you like. Don't let someone else's negative programs stop you from getting rid of yours.

7. *You may go from high enthusiasm, to completely unsure, and then back to being confident again.*

One day you may have complete belief in what the new Self-Talk says; the next day you may think it is nothing more than a few foolish words, painting a fantasy that could never come true.

As you learn what the new Self-Talk programs really sound like, and *feel* like, it is natural to wonder if they will actually work. The better the new programs sound, the harder it is for us to believe in them—at least for a while, anyway. That is because the new programs are so often the exact *opposite* of the old programs—it is no wonder the two of them are in complete conflict with each other.

The Self-Talk techniques I have recommended for you are designed to reduce that conflict; they are designed to help you get started with a minimum of doubt and anxiety, with the emphasis clearly on positive motivation instead of spending any time looking backwards into self-doubt.

If you have doubting days, that, too, is just your old programs complaining about having to leave. Just smile and stay with it. Sometimes it is hard to get rid of guests who have overstayed their welcome. But overall, the great moments, the new awareness, the fun of practicing Self-Talk, the positive changes in your own attitude, and the "better days" you start to have, will far outweigh the occasional lapses into disbelief.

Remember, you deserve to succeed, so you will.

Chapter Twenty-Five

The Second Stage Of Self-Talk : Watching It Work

Now you really start to make progress. The old programs are beginning to change, slowly at first—but you begin to see the results. You feel like you have started spring house cleaning—out with the old and in with the new—and things start to look a little better.

THE SECOND STAGE OF SELF-TALK— THE NEW PROGRAMS BEGIN TO MOVE IN TO STAY

I once gave the example of living in an apartment full of old, broken, hand-me-down furniture. The old "furniture" is the old programs that you have been living with. But you're tired of them, and you want to make some changes, so finally you decide to get rid of the old furniture, throw it all out, and never use it any more.

But we have learned that it doesn't do any good to try to get rid of the *old* furniture if you don't have some great *new* furniture to move in, in its place. That is, it doesn't work to just decide to get rid of your old programs unless you have some *better* programs to immediately replace the old ones with.

Since I first used that example, we have learned that the old furniture will never really get carried out and sent away until you *first* bring in the new furniture to replace it. Unless you *start* by bringing in plenty of new Self-Talk to replenish your "mental apartment," you will always go back out to the storage shed and bring back in the broken chair, the worn-out couch, and the tattered old rug—all of those comfortable old programs that we are so used to living with.

Our old programs, if not replaced by something better, will simply wait until they are called upon, and *instantly*, they are once again a part of our lives, looking just as unsightly and in need of repair as before.

On the other hand, when you completely redecorate your mental apartment with the new Self-Talk, you can take the old furniture out and get rid of it. You won't be needing it any longer. And that is what happens during the second stage of Self-Talk. Not only do you redecorate your mental apartment—you bring in the new furniture, and begin to get rid of the old furniture for good.

It is during this stage of Self-Talk that you start to actually *feel* the new programs taking hold. This is the time when you begin to notice changes in your habits—a tendency to change what you eat and opt for healthier menu choices, as an example. You might also notice other effects that seem to have nothing at all to do with your primary goal of losing weight or staying trim.

You may find yourself being more organized, getting places on time, if, as an example, you were not always on time before. You may notice changes in the way you are talking to other people, especially your spouse and your children and your close friends.

THIS IS WHEN STAYING WITH IT
BEGINS TO PAY OFF

Recently a single mother of three told me that she had started using Self-Talk about a year earlier. Since that time, she said, her life had changed. Her home was now in order, her kids were achieving in school, her work had improved noticeably, and she now weighed 46 pounds less than she had a year before. The only thing she and her family had done differently, she said—and she was beaming very proudly—was to start using Self-Talk.

The woman hadn't gone on another diet: she had stepped into the second stage of Self-Talk. The change in her weight alone was worth the effort it took. And there is no way to measure the value of the changes in the rest of her life.

I meet a lot of people like that now. I meet them in schools, in churches, in their businesses or in their homes—everywhere I go. I know why their stories are so encouraging. It is because they are all real people, just like you and me, and all of them are making their lives work better because they stayed with Self-Talk long enough to let the second stage take hold.

Not long ago, my wife Bonnie decided to use a special program of Self-Talk to help her maintain an important goal of her own. Over a period of time Bonnie had mastered Self-Talk and had used it to help her reach many of her goals, one of which was to get in the exact physical condition that she wanted to be in.

But now we were scheduled to do a seminar tour, and that meant we would be eating in hotel restaurants for several months. Bonnie wanted to trim down some, but she wanted especially to make sure she at least maintained her weight, if not lose a few more pounds. She decided that using Self-Talk would be the perfect "insurance" against gaining any weight on the road.

She listened to a week-by-week "refresher" program of Self-Talk tapes I often recommend to people who want to get on a good maintenance program, and she continued to listen *while* we began our travels. Bonnie is now down over thirty pounds and three dress sizes from where she was when we started the tour. She has not been on a diet a single day of that time. (That made *me* happy because it meant *I* didn't have to eat any "diet" food, either.)

That is a good picture of what can happen during stage two of Self-Talk. It doesn't mean every old program is discarded or changed for good; it means the new programs of Self-Talk are gaining strength, and beginning to take over.

IT IS NOW THAT THE SELF-TALK BEGINS TO STEP IN AND GO TO WORK ON ITS OWN

It is during stage two of Self-Talk that you begin to experience some of the new programs taking off and running on their own. These are the programs that cause other good programs you already have to work for you even harder. What's actually happening is the new Self-Talk is calling to attention the other good programs you've already got. The combination of new Self-Talk programs and the best of your old programs begin to form a team that will grow stronger and stronger the more Self-Talk practice you put in.

One of the results of this is that you will notice changes in the choices you make. You will think a moment or two longer about more of your choices, making sure they are, in fact, truly healthy choices.

During this same time you feel more in control. You exercise self-control, and you begin to see the results. Your self-esteem gets a welcome boost, and that in itself makes you feel better about yourself. And so, the cycle of positive, healthy Self-Talk, creating good habits and actions, and building even more healthy Self-Talk, takes over.

Within even a few weeks, for most people, stage two of Self-Talk is making changes, helping you get focused on your goal, and implanting great new programs.

This is the stage of Self-Talk many people thought was the *end* result. You start getting in shape, the old programs are dying out and you can feel it happen, and your attitude and your choices are clearly starting to change.

But even stage two, with all of its benefits, may actually be just the beginning. As we are learning more every day, if you stay with it now, there's still more to come.

Chapter Twenty-Six

The Final Stage Of Self-Talk : The Change

The third stage of Self-Talk takes longer to reach, but this is the most exciting and most important Self-Talk stage of all.

If the second stage of Self-Talk is the chrysalis, the third stage is the beautiful butterfly, fully grown and majestic, spreading its wings and flying into the future. This stage, for you, is the transformation, the rebirth of incredibly valuable facets of your own identity that were hidden within you—awakening parts of yourself that were good, and meaningful, and were waiting to come to life.

A MAN WHO HAD GIVEN UP HOPE

A man I met had shared his life with alcohol for over twenty years. He had fought it for years, and tried many times to quit, but continually failed. Finally, even though it was ruining his life, he gave up. He decided the best he could do would be to make the best of what he had left. To do that, he decided to get himself organized, and improve himself in any *other* area he could. So he started using Self-Talk—not for the problem with alcohol, but for the other areas of his life he *could* do something about.

Then, one day, months later, completely surprising even himself, the man *reentered* life with a clarity he had never known. Quite suddenly, with no warning, his life changed—he stopped drinking.

His "new leaf" included no alcohol, no desire to have it, and no fear. Just the strong, clear-headed confidence of a man whose old, self-destructive programs had finally been replaced with something better, and a life ahead of him he would live, completely, for the first time in years.

The man who lived that story came up to me at a seminar and told me *exactly* what Self-Talk had done for him. Self-Talk had changed his life in ways he had never even imagined. He had been listening to and practicing Self-Talk for a year or more before he awoke one day to face a new person looking at him in the mirror.

The Self-Talk he had focused on had to do with getting more organized, setting and reaching goals, and getting more in control of his life. He had *not* been using Self-Talk specifically to help him with his problem with alcohol. In fact, he had avoided even talking about that as a problem. He believed his problem with alcohol was an "impossible" problem, one he was destined to live with, and he had believed it would be with him for the rest of his life.

But meanwhile, the Self-Talk, on its own, while the man was working on something *else*, had gone to work on the *real* problem.

A WOMAN NAMED EVE

A quiet woman named Eve lost her husband just two years before his planned retirement, and many years before they were ready for him to go.

Eve's life was devastated. She had relied on their relationship for everything. Then, suddenly, she was left with her grief, no career of any kind, hardly the confidence to even go shopping alone, an empty house, a very empty life, and not a single plan for her future.

I met Eve nearly three years later. She told me that shortly after her husband died, to help her with her grief, someone had given her a copy of *"What To Say When You Talk To Your Self."* She had then attended an in-person Self-Talk training program with several of her friends in the city where she and her husband had lived.

Following that Self-Talk training seminar, Eve had continued to struggle through the mountain of difficulties the death of her husband had left her with. But she began to practice the Self-Talk techniques she had learned, and she stayed with it, mainly because she noticed that with the Self-Talk she thought more positively, and it kept her going.

But it was over a year later that almost by complete surprise, Eve suddenly began to "find" herself—and not just a return of her earlier self, either. This new Eve was more active, and more energetic. She set goals, made new friends, started a new "career" as a guidance counselor, studied French in preparation for a trip to Europe, and was not only happy, but she had started looking at life as though it had just begun.

Of special interest was what Eve told me about the *way* it had happened. "I just kept going along from day to day," she told me, "without any real sense of where I was going. A lot of the days I really don't even remember; it was all just kind of a gray time for me. But throughout it all I kept working with the Self-Talk," she said. "I don't know what I was expecting, if anything at all. I just stayed with it because it kept me going."

"Then, after all that time, one morning everything changed," Eve said. "It was like I stepped out of one picture of me and into another one. It wasn't that the grief had gone away; some of that stays. It was like someone had come in during the night, and gave me a whole new future while I was sleeping."

Eve told me about her discovery, the secret she had come to share with me. It was a story that, as I learned more and more about Self-Talk, and watched it grow in many people's lives, I had now heard many times before. "It was the Self-Talk," Eve said. "The new picture of me was a perfect *duplicate* of the new Self-Talk I had been practicing for a year and a half!"

She said, "It was doing something more important than just getting me through each day. But I didn't even know it until that day I looked in the mirror and everything had changed. The Self-Talk was getting me ready for the next twenty years of my life." And then she added, "*And I'm going for it!*"

WHAT IF YOU COULD FIND YOUR FUTURE IN THE WORDS OF SELF-TALK?

What those stories have in common with so many others I have heard during the past few years is that "something" very important happened to each of those people. And in each case, it happened on its own, and came by complete surprise—*after* they had been using Self-Talk to help them with something *else* in their lives.

This usually unexpected and somewhat remarkable third stage of Self-Talk would make every moment of practicing or listening to Self-Talk worthwhile, even if this final result were the *only* result.

But I have so often thought about how few people would ever even try Self-Talk in the first place, if they thought all Self-Talk would do for them was something that would happen down the road, months or even years from now. Even if there were, down that road, a "transformation" waiting for them, how many people would be willing to invest in it or wait for it?

It has been my experience that most people would rather invest in something they can see, right now. There isn't a lot of belief in the "transformation" business these days.

But that, too, is okay. The third stage of Self-Talk, if it has a transformation or a metamorphosis in store for you, seems to offer that extra gift free of charge. We work to achieve the first two stages of Self-Talk, and the third stage just quietly comes in on its own. We put our efforts into the two stages we can see; and the results we look for from those first two stages come soon enough so that it lets us know that practicing the Self-Talk was more than worth the effort.

THE GIFT OF SELF-TALK MAY GIVE YOU *MORE* THAN CONTROL OF YOUR WEIGHT

And so you begin.

You first become aware of your past self-talk, you practice the new Self-Talk and you begin to turn your old self-talk around. You feel the motivation and the new enthusiasm it gives you, and you look forward more optimistically as you set new goals and watch them take shape. As you continue, you not only improve your weight, your health, your attitude and your state of mind, but you begin to change some of your programs as well.

But when you start to get in control of your weight and the programs that caused the weight in the first place by changing your Self-Talk, you unleash an even greater strength within you. In time, that new strength does more than pay attention to your weight and your health; it forms a new picture of you that is stronger and more in control in every other area of your life as well.

Having to wait months or even a year or more for that new picture of you, or that new sense of confidence and purpose in your life to happen, may seem like too long a wait to make it worthwhile. But if one day you get up in the morning and something has changed, something wonderful and new has happened—go ahead: look in the mirror and see what you see.

If it happens for you, at that moment you probably won't remember about the third stage of Self-Talk, or about "transformations."

You'll be too busy getting to know the incredible person we all knew you were all along. You'll be getting ready to step away from the discarded chrysalis, spread those majestic wings toward tomorrow, and *fly*.

For more information:

For information on currently available Self-Talk Cassettes, including a special "starter set" of Self-Talk for Weight-Loss cassettes available by phone, you may contact the publisher of Self-Talk Cassettes directly at:

Telephone 1-800-982-8196

For information on "Diets Don't Work" and other books, audio or video tapes available from Dr. Bob Schwartz, contact:

Diets Don't Work Information
P.O. Box 2866
Houston, TX 77252-2866

Telephone 1-800-227-1152

DR. SHAD HELMSTETTER is the author of seven books, including the bestseller *What to Say When You Talk to Your Self*. Dr. Schwartz is the *New York Times* bestselling author of the classics *Diets Don't Work* and *Diets Still Don't Work*. Both lost over fifty pounds each more than a decade ago. Neither has gained back the weight and neither has been on a diet a single day since.

MIND MEETS BODY...
HEALTH MEETS HAPPINESS...
SPIRIT MEETS SERENITY...

In his writings, spiritual advisor Edgar Cayce counseled thousands with his extraordinary, yet practical guidance to the mind/body/spirit connection. Now, the Edgar Cayce series, based on actual readings by the renowned psychic, can provide you with insights in the search for understanding and meaning in life.

KEYS TO HEALTH: The Promise and Challenge of Holism
Eric A. Mein, M.D.
_____ 95616-9 $4.99 U.S./$5.99 CAN.

REINCARNATION: Claiming Your Past, Creating Your Future
Lynn Elwell Sparrow
_____ 95754-8 $4.99 U.S./$5.99 CAN.

DREAMS: Tonight's Answers for Tomorrow's Questions
Mark Thurston, Ph.D.
_____ 95771-8 $5.50 U.S./$6.50 CAN.

We've all been there—angry at ourselves for overeating, for our lack of willpower, for failing at yet another diet that was supposed to be the last one. But the problem is not you, it's that dieting, with its emphasis on rules and regulations, has stopped you from listening to your body. Now you can rediscover the pleasures of eating and rebuild your body image.

INTUITIVE EATING

EVELYN TRIBOLE, M.S., R.D.
AND ELYSE RESCH, M.S., R.D.